*"ARFID Avoidan   _ _...... ..1 Guide for
Parents and Carers* is an outstanding resource designed to help parents/carers understand the complexities of a diagnosis of ARFID, its consequences and treatment. This accessible guide combines clinical cases and up-to-date research. Bryant-Waugh's depth of experience working with children and families with ARFID brilliantly captures how to make sense of the everyday challenges that a diagnosis of ARFID brings to children and their families. This 'go-to' resource fills a much needed gap in providing parents/carers with strategies in supporting their child with ARFID."

Debra K. Katzman, MD, Professor of Pediatrics, Hospital for
Sick Children and University of Toronto

"This is a brilliantly written, clear, practical and engaging book by the world-expert in the field. It uniquely combines research and clinical wisdom, illustrated by multiple varied examples, to provide a comprehensive understanding of the problem and how to address it. The 5-step approach is exceptionally valuable with sequential guidance about how to enable positive change. It is essential reading for any parent or practitioner wanting to help children overcome these difficulties and is a fantastic resource that has the potential to transform lives."

Roz Shafran, Professor of Translational Psychology UCL
Great Ormond Street Institute of Child Health

"This is a long overdue guide for parents. Dr Bryant-Waugh has been a leading clinical and research expert in feeding difficulties for many years, and it is pleasing to see this wealth of experience and advice into one volume. I have no doubt it will be extremely helpful for families and children with ARFID. The suggested approaches are positive, non-blaming and focused on hope, for this is key as many children will manage and improve, but a whole family and inspiration of confidence are needed. This book provides both."

Dr Lee Hudson, Consultant Paediatrician Great
Ormond Street Hospital

ARFID Avoidant Restrictive Food Intake Disorder

ARFID Avoidant Restrictive Food Intake Disorder: A Guide for Parents and Carers is an accessible summary of a relatively recent diagnostic term. People with ARFID may show little interest in eating, eat only a very limited range of foods or may be terrified something might happen to them if they eat, such as choking or being sick. Because it has been poorly recognised and poorly understood it can be difficult to access appropriate help and difficult to know how best to manage at home.

This book covers common questions encountered by parents or carers whose child has been given a diagnosis of ARFID or who have concerns about their child. Written in simple, accessible language and illustrated with examples throughout, this book answers common questions using the most up-to-date clinical knowledge and research.

Primarily written for parents and carers of young people, *ARFID Avoidant Restrictive Food Intake Disorder* includes a wealth of practical tips and suggested strategies to equip parents and carers with the means to take positive steps towards dealing with the problems ARFID presents. It will also be relevant for family members, partners or carers of older individuals, as well as professionals seeking a useful text, which captures the full range of ARFID presentations and sets out positive management advice.

Rachel Bryant-Waugh is a Consultant Clinical Psychologist with over 30 years of experience, specialising in the study and treatment of feeding and eating disorders in children and young people. She is an internationally renowned expert with a high level of clinical and research activity in this field.

ARFID Avoidant Restrictive Food Intake Disorder

A Guide for Parents and Carers

Rachel Bryant-Waugh

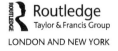

Routledge
Taylor & Francis Group

LONDON AND NEW YORK

First published 2020
by Routledge
2 Park Square, Milton Park, Abingdon, Oxon OX14 4RN

and by Routledge
52 Vanderbilt Avenue, New York, NY 10017

Routledge is an imprint of the Taylor & Francis Group, an informa business

British Library Cataloguing-in-Publication Data
A catalogue record for this book is available from the British Library

Library of Congress Cataloging-in-Publication Data
A catalog record has been requested for this book

ISBN: 978-0-367-08608-4 (hbk)
ISBN: 978-0-367-08610-7 (pbk)
ISBN: 978-0-429-02335-4 (ebk)

Typeset in Times New Roman
by Taylor & Francis Books

Printed in the UK by Severn, Gloucester on responsibly sourced paper

For Alexander, Will, Annelies and Joe, who have always helped me to keep things in perspective when it comes to parenting, children's eating, and family mealtimes.

Contents

Illustrations

Figures

Tables

Acknowledgements

With heartfelt thanks to all the families I have had the privilege to work with over the years and from whom I have learned so much. My foremost aim has long been to ensure that your stories and experiences are captured through research and writing, and used to continually shape my own clinical practice for the benefit of other families in similar situations. For all the times I have not got things right, or have misunderstood, I apologise.

Many thanks to my trusty 'critical friends' for help with reading the manuscript through and making suggestions for clarifications and changes to make the text more readable and easier to follow.

Preface

Above all else, this book is intended to be useful; to be read, dipped into, returned to, or used to open a conversation, as fits the reader's preferences, circumstances or requirements. It aims to provide an update on the current state of knowledge about ARFID in clear language, free of jargon and bias. It covers questions frequently asked by parents or carers whose child has been given a diagnosis of ARFID as well as by those who have concerns that their child may be showing signs of this disorder. In order to illustrate situations in a meaningful way, examples of the wide range of different types of difficulty encountered by those affected by avoidant and restrictive eating behaviours are woven through the text.

Throughout the book, the personal and possessive pronouns 'they', 'them', 'their' are used in relation to 'child', rather than 'he/she', 'him/her', 'his/hers', to include all children whatever their sex or gender. The term 'child' is used here to refer to infants, children, and young people up to the age of 18 years. When 'your child' is referred to, this could therefore include teenage offspring. The intention is to be as inclusive as possible; after all ARFID occurs across this age range and into adulthood. The term 'parents' is sometimes used alone and sometimes in conjunction with 'carers'. When used alone it usually refers to anyone in a primary parenting role, whether they are a biological parent, or other primary care-giver. Finally, the words 'we' and 'our' are predominantly used to refer to people in general, rather than to clinicians, scientists, or any other single group. The author is a mental health practitioner and academic, but also a parent, daughter, partner, and friend. A distinction between 'us' (clinicians, scientists) and 'you'/'them' (parents/carers) seems artificial and unnecessary. It also goes against the collaborative style of working, recommended in this book, which is based on sharing knowledge and integrating perspectives.

A number of themes run throughout the text, which have been used to provide structure and aid understanding. These include the concept of ARFID being an 'umbrella' diagnosis; that is, the important fact that ARFID in one person does not necessarily look identical to ARFID in another. Not only does it not necessarily take the same form, it may have arisen from a completely different set of circumstances. The need to explore the specific contributing and maintaining factors for each individual is emphasised; only then can attempts to address difficulties be appropriately targeted and managed. This requirement to tailor approaches to support any one child and family means that not everything in this book will resonate with any one reader. The breadth of ARFID presentations requires a wide ranging discussion; as a consequence it is likely that not everything will be relevant to everyone.

Another thread running through the book is reference to one or more of what are referred to here as six core 'C factors'. These six 'C factors' are: *characteristics; correlates; causes; consequences; care*; and *course*. They are put forward as aspects of ARFID that are central to our understanding of its development and its features, as well as to the strategies recommended to try to address difficulties and facilitate change. At present, further research is needed across all six of these areas, in order to improve knowledge and management of ARFID.

This book is therefore intended as a reliable, go-to source of straightforward practical advice and suggestions, aimed at increasing knowledge through giving an up-to-date account of the state of the field in plain, everyday language. It represents a synthesis and summary of clinical expertise and research evidence to date. It has been written primarily for parents and carers of children and young people with ARFID. It could, however, also be relevant for family members, partners, or carers of older individuals, as ARFID occurs in people of all ages. Hopefully, the book will also prove to be relevant to professionals as an easy-to-read text which captures the full range of ARFID presentations and sets out positive management advice.

Rachel Bryant-Waugh
January 2019

Glossary

aetiology	a term that is often used in medical texts to mean the causes of a condition or disease
anaemia	a medical condition with low red blood cell count; iron deficiency anaemia is often caused by insufficient iron in the diet and characterised by tiredness, weakness, and lack of energy
anorexia nervosa	a formal diagnostic term for an eating disorder characterised by extreme restriction of food intake driven by concerns about weight and/or shape; individuals with anorexia nervosa are typically low in weight and will avoid gaining weight
anti-histamine	a type of medication developed principally to manage allergic conditions, through dampening the body's response to histamine which causes the reaction
anti-psychotic	a type of medication developed principally to manage psychotic disorders, such as schizophrenia and bipolar disorder, but since used to treat a number of other non-psychotic disorders
Asperger's syndrome	a term previously used to denote a type of autism spectrum disorder, typically characterised by high levels of motor activity and specific interests as well as difficulties in interaction, but with less speech delay and difficulty than other types of autism

attention deficit hyperactivity disorder (ADHD)	a formal diagnostic term for a condition that is characterised by difficulties with attention, often with impulsivity and high levels of activity
autism spectrum disorder (ASD)	a formal diagnostic term for a range of conditions that affect a person's interactions with others, communication, interests, and behaviour; ASD previously included Asperger's syndrome
avidity	a descriptive term sometimes used in relation to food which captures enthusiasm to eat; this in turn may rest on the presence of a range of factors, including hunger, liking of the food in question, and readiness to eat
behavioural feeding problems	a term sometimes used to differentiate feeding and eating difficulties that stem from emotional, psychological or behavioural factors, rather than feeding and eating difficulties with a primary medical cause
binge eating disorder	a formal diagnostic term for an eating disorder characterised by episodes of eating accompanied by a sense of loss of control and distress; unlike bulimia nervosa this is not followed by behaviour intended to counteract the effects of eating, such as vomiting or misusing laxatives so that many individuals with this form of eating disorder are at a high weight
biopsychosocial model	a model put forward to understand health as an interplay of biological, psychological, and social factors
bulimia nervosa	a formal diagnostic term for an eating disorder characterised by episodes of eating accompanied by a sense of loss of control, followed by behaviour intended to counteract the effects of eating, such as vomiting or misusing laxatives
calories	units of energy stored in food and needed to maintain weight and growth

caseness	a term used to denote whether a person's symptoms meet diagnostic criteria for a particular condition or disorder
cognitive behavioural therapy	a well-established form of psychological treatment where a focus is placed on understanding and working to change thoughts, beliefs, and behaviours that are causing difficulty for the individual and are related to distress or impairment to daily functioning
correlates	factors that tend to co-occur and where one thing has a relationship with or influences another
course	the term often used to describe the path an illness or condition takes over time
cyproheptadine	a type of medicine in the class of anti-histamines, originally developed primarily for use in the treatment of allergies to limit the body's allergic response; cyproheptadine has since been shown to be helpful in some patients with a range of other conditions
differential diagnosis/ diagnoses	a term given to denote the process a clinician will go through, usually when assessing a patient to arrive at a diagnosis, which involves giving consideration to other possible diagnoses that may share some of the reported symptoms
DSM-IV	the fourth edition of the Diagnostic and Statistical Manual of Mental Disorders; the diagnostic and classification system of the American Psychiatric Association; this version has been replaced by DSM-5
DSM-5	the fifth edition of the Diagnostic and Statistical Manual of Mental Disorders; the diagnostic and classification system of the American Psychiatric Association; this is the current manual
dysphagia	a formal term used to describe swallowing difficulties that result from a range of medical conditions and oral-motor problems

eating disorder not otherwise specified (EDNOS)	a formal diagnostic term in DSM-IV, now no longer in use, to describe individuals who had clinically significant forms of eating disturbance but who did not meet full diagnostic criteria for anorexia nervosa or bulimia nervosa; EDNOS, one of the eating disorders, included a varied group of difficulties, including binge eating disorder and likely to have included some individuals with ARFID
enteral feeding	often used as another name for tube feeding; technically enteral feeding includes any type of feeding that goes through the intestine, either via the mouth and throat, or via a tube (nasogastric or gastrostomy); it can be distinguished from parenteral feeding, which is when a person is fed via another route, such as through a drip into the blood stream
epipen	a pre-loaded syringe type of device that can be used by an individual in the case of an extreme allergic reaction to inject an appropriate dose of medication to dampen the response
evidence-based practice	a term used to describe clinical practice, to include specific procedures, interventions and treatments, that are based on available evidence that they are safe and effective
extreme picky eating	a descriptive term used to describe eating behaviour characterised by the individual only accepting a very narrow range of foods, to an extent that is more extreme than the sort of picky eating that might normally be seen; unlike 'normal' picky eating, extreme picky eating tends to persist and can be associated with impairment to health and daily functioning
faltering growth	a term used to describe children with very low weight, or who are failing to maintain an expected rate of growth and/or weight, previously often referred to as 'failure to thrive'

feeding disorder of infancy or early childhood	a formal diagnostic term applicable to children whose feeding difficulties started before the age of six years, characterised by an inability to take in enough food to maintain weight and grow normally; this diagnosis has been replaced and extended with the introduction of ARFID
food avoidance emotional disorder (FAED)	a descriptive term used to describe an eating difficulty characterised by low interest in eating, often in the context of generalised emotional distress; individuals with FAED tend to struggle to eat an adequate amount, resulting in loss of weight
food neophobia	a descriptive term used to describe an extreme fear (phobia) of new (neo) foods which typically leads to extreme caution, avoidance or refusal in relation to trying any foods outside the individual's usual range of foods eaten
food phobia	a general term used to describe a general fear of food that is extreme which may lead to avoidance of eating or restriction of food intake
functional dysphagia	a descriptive term previously used to describe a condition characterised by the individual experiencing difficulties swallowing, despite there being no medical evidence for this; it may be related to a fear of choking or a sense of having a lump in the throat
gastrostomy tube	a feeding tube that has been inserted through the stomach wall and allows feed to go directly into the stomach; such a tube may be used when the individual is unable to eat enough by mouth or has difficulty swallowing
ICD-11	The International Classification of Diseases – Eleventh edition (ICD-11) is an updated version of the classification system developed by the World Health Organization and used throughout the world; it provides descriptions and diagnostic criteria for a wide range of medical conditions as well as mental and behavioural disorders

infantile anorexia	a descriptive term used to describe infants and young children who appear to have low appetite; such children often struggle to gain weight and may become malnourished
jejunum	the middle part of the small intestine where most of the nutrients from food are absorbed
macronutrients	essential constituents of the diet, made up of a number of types of food needed in relatively large amounts and necessary to maintain good health and functioning; carbohydrates, proteins, fruit, and vegetables are examples of essential micronutrients
micronutrients	essential constituents of the diet, usually only needed in small amounts, but necessary to maintain good health and functioning; vitamins and minerals are examples of essential micronutrients
modifiable risk factors	factors that raise an individual's likelihood of developing a specific condition or disease that can in theory be altered; these typically include factors such diet, exercise, certain lifestyle choices such as smoking, alcohol use, and other behaviours known to have adverse consequences for health
nasogastric tube	a flexible type of feeding tube that is inserted up through the nose and then goes down the oesophagus into the stomach; this may be used in individuals who are acutely malnourished and unable to take enough food orally
non-modifiable risk factors	factors that raise an individual's likelihood of developing a specific condition or disease that cannot be altered; these typically include factors such as age, sex, ethnicity, genetic make-up, family history
obsessive compulsive disorder (OCD)	a condition, classified as a psychiatric or mental disorder, characterised by obsessions (often in the form of intrusive, unwanted thoughts) and compulsions (usually in the form of repeated behaviours) that interfere with a person's day-to-day functioning and are associated with distress

olanzapine	a type of medicine in the class of anti-psychotics, originally developed primarily for use in the treatment of schizophrenia and bipolar disorder; it has since been used in a wider range of mental disorders with some evidence of positive effect in certain groups of patients
orthorexia	a descriptive term rather than a formal diagnosis, used to describe a condition characterised by the individual going to extreme lengths to avoid foods that they consider to be unhealthy; in its extreme form, such individuals can exclude a wide range of foods so that they become severely nutritionally compromised
patient-centred care	a term used to describe an approach to health care design and delivery that takes account of patients' views, wishes, and preferences; decision making about care involves the input of the patient, who should be provided with appropriate information to enable informed choices to be made
PEG (Percutaneous Endoscopic Gastrostomy)	a type of medical procedure where a feeding tube is passed through the stomach wall directly into the stomach; 'percutaneous' means through the skin, 'endoscopic' means that an endoscope, or flexible tube, is used to complete the procedure rather than surgery; and 'gastrostomy' means tube into the stomach.
PEG-J (Percutaneous Endoscopic Gastro-Jejunostomy, or Percutaneous Endoscopic Transgastric Jejunostomy)	as with a PEG, this is a similar type of medical procedure but in a PEG-J the tube goes into the jejunum rather than the stomach; sometimes this is done with an extension to a PEG and sometimes the tube is placed directly in the jejunum

pica | a condition, classified as a psychiatric or mental disorder, that involves the person eating non-food items, such as dirt, chalk, or cloth

randomised controlled trial (RCT) | a type of research study, generally considered to be of high quality, that corrects for factors that might be influencing the findings; RCT studies are often used to test different types of treatment

rickets | a medical condition that typically results from long-standing inadequate intake of specific nutrients in the diet, including vitamin D or calcium; it is characterised by weak bones and skeletal deformities

rumination disorder | a condition, classified as a psychiatric or mental disorder, that involves the person bringing previously eaten food back up into the mouth through regurgitation; the food is typically re-chewed and may be re-swallowed or spat out; this can have the function of helping to regulate emotions

scurvy | a medical disease caused by insufficient vitamin C in the diet, typically accompanied by tiredness, feeling weak and aches and pains, particularly in the legs

selective eating disorder | a term previously used to describe individuals accepting only a limited range of foods, usually on the basis of their sensory properties, including texture, taste, and appearance

sensory diet | an individualised programme, usually drawn up by an occupational therapist, that can help a person manage everyday sensory input and remain more focussed and calm

sensory food aversion | a term used by some to describe the avoidance of certain foods on the basis of their sensory properties; such foods typically evoke disgust in the individual concerned

stunting | a medical term with various formal definitions, often used to describe a chronic form of malnutrition which results in slowed growth in childhood, so that children end up much smaller than their peers; stunting can also occur for non-nutritional reasons in some individuals tube weaning   the process of reducing dependency on tube feeds through increasing oral food and fluid intake; amounts of feed are generally reduced as the individual accepts more by mouth, until tube feeding is no longer needed

wasting   a medical term with various formal definitions, used to describe an acute form of malnutrition in people who have typically lost a lot of weight and have lost muscle tissue and fat; in children this may include very underweight children who have been unable to gain weight

Introduction

This is a book about ARFID – perhaps not a name to trip off the tongue and indeed one that many people have never even heard of. This is perhaps not entirely surprising given that ARFID, or 'avoidant/restrictive food intake disorder', was first introduced as a term as recently as 2013. Before then, although ARFID did not exist as a formal diagnosis or formally recognised condition, the eating difficulties it covers certainly did. These were known by a large range of different names which included 'feeding disorder', 'selective eating disorder', 'food neophobia', 'functional dysphagia', 'infantile anorexia', 'sensory food aversion', 'extreme picky eating', 'food avoidance emotional disorder', 'food phobia', 'behavioural feeding problems', and many more. All these different names meant slightly different things to different people, which in turn meant that developments in treatment did not really progress as well as they might have otherwise. It was a bit like being in a room full of people trying to talk about a common topic, but all speaking different languages. In such a situation, there may be a shared understanding of a few words, but communication between individuals can only take place in a very simple way. We know that the best research, which is so needed to underpin positive changes in health care, relies on collaboration and being able to replicate the results of treatment trials. If there is poor agreement, or if there are variations in understanding about what you are talking about in the first place, you can see the problem!

If you are a parent, you may have started reading this book because your child, or a child in your wider family, has eating habits that are causing you concern. They may be struggling to eat a sufficient amount or an adequate range of foods and you want to find out more. You may be a teacher, a child-care worker, or a family friend with worries about a child you know, or you may be a health-care professional seeing children and their families in a clinic setting. Whoever you are, you may have searched on the Internet for more information about eating difficulties and in doing so, come across ARFID. Alternatively, you may have heard about ARFID from colleagues, friends or relatives. One thing may well have struck you – there seems to be a fair amount of confusion and difference of opinion about what it is and how it can best be managed. Again, perhaps this is not entirely surprising given its recent introduction and the preceding muddle of terms, but confusion and differences of opinion can be far from helpful if you need reliable, up-to-date information and advice. That is where this book about ARFID comes in. Its content is based in part on the questions, concerns, insights, challenges, and successes of many families who have first-hand experience of ARFID. My work over many years has brought me together with these families and one of my responsibilities to them has been to ensure that their stories and experiences are shared. The text is also informed by experience derived from clinical practice and research to date, which has focussed on ARFID and restrictive eating difficulties. The aim of the book is to provide information to help with uncertainty, to foster hope and understanding, and to relieve some of the worry and distress that may accompany having a child with ARFID.

The text is structured around common questions, asked by many parents. What is ARFID exactly? Who can develop it, and why? What happens to someone who has ARFID? Can it be treated and will it ever go away? Is it dangerous? What are the immediate and longer-term implications for health? What can I do? What about the future? Is someone with ARFID likely to develop all sorts of other problems? One of the themes running through the book is the importance of what are referred to here as the core 'C factors'. These are illustrated in Figure 0.1 below. They include important aspects of ARFID, namely, *Character-istics* (discussed in Chapter 1 – What is ARFID?); *Correlates*, or

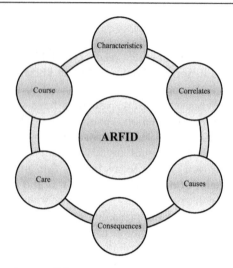

Figure 0.1 The six core C factors

things that tend to go with having ARFID (discussed in Chapter 2 – Who can develop ARFID?); *Causes* (discussed in Chapter 3 – Why does someone develop ARFID?); *Consequences* (discussed in Chapter 4 – What are the consequences of having ARFID?); *Care* (discussed in Chapter 5 – What can I do?, and in Chapter 6 – What is the best treatment for ARFID?); and *Course* (discussed in Chapter 7 – What about the future?). The 'C factors' certainly all need further exploration if we are to improve our knowledge of ARFID, and in particular if we are to be able to know how best to match different treatment approaches to different individuals.

Most professionals delivering health-care related interventions are expected to engage in 'evidence-based practice'. In essence this means that any decisions about how best to manage or treat a condition should be based on the best available evidence at the time. This requires clinicians to be informed about current knowledge and research developments in their field of practice and to use this knowledge in an appropriate and relevant manner in their interactions with the people they see in clinical settings. There are a number of different definitions of evidence-based practice, but one that seems particularly helpful, and has been widely adopted, is the one first set out by David Sackett and his colleagues back in the 1990s. This proposes that there are three important components to consider equally in the delivery of evidence-based care (Sackett et al. 1996; Sackett et al. 2000):

- best available evidence from systematic research (that is, research that is clinically relevant and has been carried out using sound methods)
- knowledge derived from clinical expertise (that is, the experience of the clinician, their skills and the training and education they have received)
- patient values (that is, the person's own personal preferences, unique concerns, expectations and values)

The outcome of careful and equal consideration of these three components needs to be integrated to arrive at a plan for the best way forward for any one individual. We will return to this model of evidence-based practice in more detail in Chapter 6, when we discuss *care*. However, for now perhaps you might agree that this approach seems highly relevant when we are thinking about evidence-based care for ARFID. Systematic research is still relatively limited as the field is new, although a number of promising studies are underway and the results should helpfully inform practice. On the other hand, there is considerable clinical expertise in relation to types of eating difficulty that previously might have been called different names, but are now included in the definition of ARFID. Most important of all, 'patient values' is key; so many parents describe concerns about their child's eating that are real and pressing, but do not appear to have been heard by those they have approached for help. It is extremely important to attend to this aspect of the triad of a comprehensive evidence-based practice approach, as without doing so, care may be compromised.

This book, ARFID: *A Guide for Parents and Carers*, is therefore set against a changing background. It does not set out to be the last word on the subject; far from it, it is to be hoped that over the coming years it will be possible to take significant steps forward, so that together we can all provide effective support and input at the earliest opportunity. Before we proceed through the questions outlined above, and a consideration of our core C factors, it seems sensible to start at the beginning.

Avoidant/restrictive food intake disorder, or ARFID, made its first appearance as we have seen, in 2013. It was included as one of the Feeding and Eating Disorders in the diagnostic manual of the American Psychiatric Association, called the DSM-5, which was published that year (American Psychiatric Association 2013). 'DSM' stands for *Diagnostic and Statistical Manual*, here pertaining to clinical presentations that are designated 'mental disorders'. The number '5' denotes that this is the fifth edition of the American Psychiatric Association's manual. The reason there have been a number of editions is because diagnostic categories are not fixed. They generally represent what is regarded as the best way to capture and represent recognisable patterns of mental distress and behavioural difficulties that people seek help for, or present in clinical settings. Given that the first edition was published back in 1952, shortly after the end of World War II, with over half a century of research in the intervening period, it is perhaps not surprising that the original classification system has undergone a number of updates and revisions.

So how did ARFID make its way into DSM-5? The quick answer is on the basis of clinical and research evidence available at the time. However, to understand this better, we need to take a step back to the situation at the time the lengthy revision process started. The research agenda that formed part of the preparations for DSM-5 was drawn up between 1999 and 2002. At this time, DSM-IV (the fourth edition of the diagnostic manual, which was first published in 1994) was in general use to define and diagnose mental disorders. In DSM-IV, the section on 'Eating Disorders' included three main diagnostic categories: 'anorexia nervosa', 'bulimia nervosa', and a third catch-all category called 'eating disorder not otherwise specified' (commonly referred to as EDNOS). DSM-IV also included a separate section on 'Feeding Disorders', which formed part of a chapter called 'Disorders Usually First Diagnosed in Infancy, Childhood, or Adolescence'. As with the eating disorders section, this feeding disorders section also included three diagnostic categories: 'pica', 'rumination disorder', and 'feeding disorder of infancy or early childhood' (see

Glossary for brief descriptions). The definition of the latter specified that the feeding problem had to have been present before the individual reached the age of 6 years, and feeding difficulties had to be accompanied by low weight. If you are familiar with ARFID, it won't be hard to spot the problem with this situation. What diagnosis would be appropriate for a teenager with avoidant or restrictive eating that is clearly distinguishable from anorexia nervosa? What term would you use for an eight-year-old who develops serious problems with food intake following a gagging or choking incident? What about someone who has always been very selective about what they will eat and has worryingly poor nutrition, but isn't underweight? Here was an unfortunate example of a relatively poor fit between available diagnostic categories and the real difficulties that people experienced. This mismatch between real life problems and available diagnostic categories was recognised as being a particular issue for the types of eating difficulty that many children were being seen for, but it was also recognised as a problem for some adults who similarly 'didn't fit'. Many of these individuals' difficulties could not be accounted for by an underlying medical condition and were primarily driven by emotional or behavioural difficulties. They were usually associated with distress and significant impairment to health, development, and everyday functioning. Such individuals, who we now describe as having ARFID, were variously given diagnoses of 'EDNOS', 'feeding disorder of infancy or early childhood', a question mark, or worse still, dismissed as not having a real problem. Such a situation was clearly extremely unhelpful and unsatisfactory in terms of people being able to access appropriate care.

Fortunately, following five years of research conferences (between 2003 and 2008) as well as five years of scrutiny of all available relevant research and clinical evidence (between 2007 and 2012), it was possible to arrive at some conclusions. The proposal was put forward that ARFID should replace 'feeding disorder of infancy or early childhood', and that its reach should be extended to encompass significant impairment related to avoidant and restrictive food intake in individuals of any age. It was suggested that ARFID should be understood as not solely a children's problem, but one that can also occur in adolescents and adults. Furthermore, it was proposed that ARFID is not necessarily characterised by low weight; some people with ARFID may indeed have very low weight, and children with the condition may have growth delay, but not all will, with many being normal weight or having higher than normal weight. The proposals for the definition of ARFID were then discussed and debated by a number of other committees, both internal and external to the American Psychiatric Association and the process of diagnostic revision. The proposals were eventually accepted on the strength of the evidence supporting the case for ARFID. The condition, with its proposed definition, therefore replaced and extended the old feeding disorder diagnosis which has now disappeared as a category in the current classification scheme.

You may well wonder if all of this matters if you are not American or seen by American health-care professionals. The answer is yes, because alongside the American Psychiatric Association's classification system is a much bigger and more comprehensive system of classifying all diseases and health problems, including those relating to both physical and mental health. This is the International Classification of Diseases, or ICD, which is the international standard of the World Health Organization. The 10th edition of the ICD system, originally endorsed in 1990 and used around the world since 1994, was also in need of an update. Very early on in the revision timelines, both the World Health Organization and the American Psychiatric Association made an agreement to co-ordinate effort as much as possible. After all, both were mining the same body of evidence to inform change. The reach of the ICD system is truly global as almost all countries in the world are member states of the World Health Organization. The ICD is used as an international standard for defining and reporting diseases and health conditions, allowing countries around the world to compare and share health information using a common language. ICD-11 (the 11th edition of the ICD system, World Health Organization 2018) was released to member states in June 2018, pending endorsement in 2019, with health reporting using the revised system due to commence in 2022. The ICD section on 'Feeding and Eating Disorders' is broadly consistent with the revised DSM diagnoses and definitions, including the addition of ARFID. It has therefore been comprehensively accepted that ARFID occurs around the world, in people of all ages and from a range of different cultures. At this stage it seems very likely that it will become a globally relevant term.

In conclusion therefore, ARFID is a formally recognised, evidence-informed term. It is not a 'made-up' problem, nor something that does not warrant our attention and ongoing attempts to understand and manage better. It is certainly the case that there is a long way to go in relation to early and reliable identification of ARFID, and it undoubtedly remains relatively poorly understood. This can mean that people struggle to access the right care and that family members are left battling their own mounting concern over their child or loved one. The way ARFID is defined and understood may well change as knowledge increases. In the future, its name may even be changed if there is incontrovertible evidence pointing in a particular direction. For now though, those three cornerstones of evidence-based practice – research evidence; clinical expertise; patient values – should also be the three cornerstones of approaches to generating new evidence. All are equally important.

We are ready now, having considered where ARFID has come from, to begin to work through our questions.

Chapter 1

What is ARFID?

What is ARFID exactly? What are its key features? Is it always the same, irrespective of who has it? In this chapter we will discuss the *characteristics* of ARFID, in which we will consider the distinctive nature and essential features of ARFID. It will cover the definition and diagnostic criteria for ARFID in some detail, as well as give examples of how different aspects of ARFID are manifested in everyday life. As this book is primarily intended for parents and carers of children under the age of 18 years, individuals in this age range will be used in the examples. However, do remember that this diagnosis can in theory be given to a person of any age, so that some of the content of the examples might apply to adults with ARFID as well. It is helpful to be fully informed about what ARFID is and what it is not, both in terms of your own understanding of the nature and extent of your child's difficulties, but also so that you can clearly describe specific areas of difficulty and why these are causing you concern.

If you read the chapter right through, the idea is that should you need to, you will be able to calmly explain that no, ARFID is not the same as normal picky or faddy eating. So many parents and carers describe professionals batting away their concerns with 'advice', such as 'No need to worry, he'll grow out of it', or 'Maybe if you were a bit firmer at mealtimes, it would help', or 'You just need to make sure she eats more fruit/vegetables/protein/ dairy / [or some food you know your child is less likely to eat than to fly to the moon and back]'. Friends and relatives may also not be the pillars of support you hope they will be. On describing the difficulties they are facing to those close to them, many parents report being told things like 'Oh yes, mine is just the same, I can't get her to eat courgettes at all...', or 'Let me have him for the weekend, we'll soon sort this out', or 'You've always been too soft with them'. Mostly, such suggestions and comments are not intended to be deliberately hurtful or unhelpful, and are for the most part likely to be borne out of a simple lack of knowledge and understanding about ARFID. Being well-informed yourself is the first step in standing your ground, helping others to understand, and doing your best as a parent to ensure your child's needs are met.

Let's start with the formal definition of ARFID. As already mentioned, the American Psychiatric Association was the first to put forward diagnostic criteria for ARFID in DSM-5 (APA 2013). In this system, there are four main requirements that have to be met before it would be appropriate for a clinician to give a formal diagnosis. The first is the most detailed and we will look at this carefully. The other three requirements that need to be met are known as 'exclusion criteria'. This means that they cover things that need to be ruled out, that is, things that are clearly not present. If one or more of these three exclusion criteria is identified, then the person would not be given an ARFID diagnosis.

The first requirement lies in the name ARFID, which as we have seen stands for avoidant/restrictive food intake disorder. There should therefore clearly be a disturbance of feeding or eating, characterised by avoidance or restriction of food intake. This disturbance may be driven by one or more of a number of different factors. In DSM-5, three examples are given, based on well-described and well-documented clinical presentations. The first example is that the avoidance or restriction may stem from a lack of interest; the second example is that it may stem from sensory-based avoidance; and the third example is that it may stem from concern about possible aversive consequences of eating. We will take a closer look at each of these factors, which may be driving the avoidance or restriction of food intake, in turn.

Lack of interest may be present either in relation to eating or in relation to food in general. Some people find it difficult to make time to eat or to remember to eat, either because they are fully engaged in doing more interesting things, or because they simply do not seem to have a very good sense of hunger and appetite. We will look at some of the possible reasons behind this apparent lack of interest in later chapters when we consider *correlates* (Chapter 2: Who can develop ARFID?) and *causes* (Chapter 3: Why does someone develop ARFID?). Sometimes low interest seems related to the individual experiencing eating as a chore, or simply not deriving pleasure or satisfaction from food. This can be hard for many of us to understand; mostly, we are very aware when we are hungry and most of us do experience some pleasure and satisfaction in eating, particularly our favourite foods. Solly's eating difficulties are an example of low interest in food and eating being a main driver for his restricted intake. He would take a very long time over his meals, often 'pouching' food in his cheeks, which is a behaviour often seen in children who are not particularly motivated to eat.

Solly is a six-year-old boy who lives with his parents and younger brother. He is a slight child who looks tired and underweight. His parents describe him as a polite boy who is quite quiet at home and at school. Solly likes to draw and colour, and can spend long periods amusing himself playing with his cars. At school, he is said to be well-behaved and does not cause his teacher any trouble. She has noticed that he is rather shy and reticent, rarely putting up his hand and happy to be on his own in the playground.

Solly's feeding had been difficult from the start. He vomited a great deal from the start and became very unwell. It took a while before his difficulty was diagnosed as pyloric stenosis (a condition in which food or, as here, fluid is prevented from passing normally through the stomach into the small intestine). This was successfully treated by surgery but unfortunately Solly then came down with a nasty chest infection and again struggled to feed. A nasogastric tube was inserted and he stayed in hospital for a while with his mother, who was understandably very worried about him. Over time, she was able to encourage him to take milk and soft foods by mouth and eventually the nasogastric tube was removed. When they attended the clinic with Solly now six years of age, his mother described it as always having been hard work trying to get him to take enough. She felt that he had never been that interested in eating.

Solly struggles with his health on and off, particularly in the winter, being prone to catching minor coughs and colds. When unwell with these, his eating tends to deteriorate and his weight gain overall is only just tracking the lower centiles on his weight chart. He has no other significant medical conditions of note.

Solly's parents describe trying to get him to eat enough as requiring a lot of effort. He will often put off coming to the table, asking to be allowed to finish playing, or to complete a colouring picture. When at the table he is a very slow eater, often chewing a mouthful for a very long time and sometimes holding food in his cheeks. His mother said that she often has to remind him to swallow so that he will move on to the next mouthful. They are worried that as he grows older he won't eat enough to keep himself healthy. The family doctor has told them that there is nothing physically wrong with Solly, he just doesn't seem interested in eating.

The second example of what might be driving the avoidance or restriction of food intake is that it may be linked to the sensory characteristics of food and the individual's particular response to these. Our senses include touch, sight, hearing, smell and taste. In relation to the sensory properties of food, as well as its taste and smell, these include its texture, temperature, appearance, colour, and the noise it makes when we eat it. People with ARFID may only eat foods of a particular texture, for example only smooth foods, or only crunchy foods. They might find certain textures extremely off-putting, to the extent that they experience disgust, and will avoid these. Mixed texture foods may be refused outright as the tongue and mouth are required to manage a number of different textures simultaneously. Yoghurt or orange juice with bits in, or a sandwich with chicken, mayonnaise and lettuce, are examples of mixed texture foods. Foods that have touched other foods may be rejected as texture has been affected. A roast potato that has had some gravy on one corner or a fish finger with a small amount of baked bean sauce on one end may be completely refused. There can be a high ability to detect even very slight changes in texture, leading to refusal; a chip is too crispy, a piece of toast is too floppy. Some people will only eat foods at a specific temperature; only straight out the fridge, or only foods at room temperature, never having eaten anything warm or hot. Others will refuse anything that does not look right to them; a black mark on a crisp, a broken biscuit, or an unevenly shaped piece of breakfast cereal. Many have a strong preference for preferred foods to be cut or presented in a certain way. If it does not look right it will not be eaten. Colour preferences may also be present, with the most common ARFID diet being the so-called 'beige diet'. This may include things like biscuits, bread, crisps, potatoes – usually high carbohydrate foods, but all a bland colour. It can be difficult to ascertain if this truly avoidance on the basis of colour, as foods of other colours such as red and green generally have stronger flavours. Beige foods generally tend to be less challenging in terms of palatability. However, it is certainly the case that if you present a true 'beige-eater' with a food of a different colour, this will usually be refused on sight. Some people will describe rejecting food because of the noise it makes when they bite or chew it, or when others eat these foods, preferring to stick to softer foods that do not cause distress in this way. Sensitivity to smell and taste is often extreme; many people with ARFID can be thought of as 'super-sensers' or 'super-tasters'. They can detect the tiniest variations in taste which makes trying to sneak something into their preferred meals perilous (see further Chapter 5: What can I do?). They may avoid certain environments, like the school dining hall or even family mealtimes because they can't manage the smell of food and some will carefully smell everything before they put it near their mouth. Kai's story is not untypical.

Kai is eight years old. He is an only child who lives with his mother and grandparents. Kai's father is not present in his life; his parents were not in a relationship when his mother became pregnant and she now has no contact with his father. Kai is described as a stubborn child who knows what he likes and prefers to be in charge. He is a much loved child and is particularly attached to his grandfather, who dotes on him. Kai's mother finds his behaviour difficult to manage at times as he is so strong willed. Kai is quite a big child for his age and there is no concern about his weight or growth.

Kai is very sensitive to smell and will often comment on the smell of something. This can be anything and anywhere and is not restricted to food. Kai's mother said that at times this can be embarrassing, giving examples of Kai making loud comments about not liking how somebody smelt on the bus, and complaining about the smell of another child's house when invited to play. He wasn't invited again. His mother and grandparents have tried to make a positive thing of this by telling Kai that he is like a police sniffer dog. Kai would like to be a policeman when he is older and so is not offended by this. He thinks his 'sniffing powers' might come in handy.

Kai's mother and grandmother describe increasing difficulty with making sure he is eating properly. Kai puts everything to his nose to smell it before eating it. He will often put something to one side saying it does not smell right. He tends to like bland foods and eats a lot of carbohydrates. Kai's mother said she has had to stop cooking certain things for herself and her parents because Kai complains so much about the smell. The family is unable to go out to eat in all but one pizza restaurant as Kai will complain about the smell of cooking or other people's food.

This has also been a problem at school. Initially, when Kai started in the Reception class, he took in a packed lunch and was allowed to sit away from the dining hall to eat it. He is now eight years old and his teachers feel he should be integrating more with his peers. They have noted that his social interactions are already quite limited. This, combined with a very limited diet, is causing his mother a great deal of concern.

The third example of what might be driving the avoidance or restriction of food intake seen in ARFID, is that it may be related to a concern about unpleasant or feared consequences of eating, for example, thinking 'if I eat this, something bad is going to happen'. The something bad could be related to a fear of vomiting or choking, worry that it will lead to nausea, discomfort or abdominal pain, or simply a worry that I won't like it. In your quest to find out more about ARFID, you may have come across the terms 'neophobia' or 'food neophobia'. This simply means a fear (phobia) of new (neo) foods. When you talk to some people about why they won't try things outside their comfort zone, some will be able to state clearly what the reason is. However, many will struggle to come up with anything specific and will usually end up concluding that the possibility that they won't like it is sufficient to put them off completely. Food neophobia can in this way be considered an example of avoidance driven by concern about aversive consequences. Other examples of avoidance of food intake stemming from fear or concern, can be found in those people who may have been frightened by an aversive experience (for example, a choking incident, such as in Emmie's case below), or those who have had a medical condition associated with discomfort, such as in Jake's case (also below).

> Emmie, aged nine, had been excited to go to the cinema with her mother and best friend Layla. The girls had asked to see a film their classmates had been talking about. However, the day before the planned trip, one child had said that the film had a very scary part and Emmie had been worried about this. Emmie usually felt braver after talking with her father in particular, when she voiced any worries and fears. On this occasion he was away on business, and so she came down to talk to her mother when she struggled to get off to sleep. She never really liked it when her father was away and although she felt somewhat reassured by her mother, she continued to worry that the film would be very scary.
>
> On the day, Emmie seemed happy to see Layla and they settled into their seats, each with a bag of sweets. All seemed to be fine, until at one point in the film there was an unexpected bang, which caused Emmie to inhale and a sweet to go down the wrong way. She started to retch and panic and her mother rushed her to the door of the cinema with an upset

Layla in tow. Emmie coughed up the sweet as they reached the door and started crying loudly. This made Layla cry as well and Emmie's mother to become somewhat cross about the fuss. Emmie was clearly terrified and refused to go into the cinema saying that she had nearly died. After trying for a while, Emmie's mother gave up and took both girls home.

Over the subsequent weeks Emmie displayed significant and mounting anxiety. In particular she was initially very on edge at mealtimes, paying attention to every sound and jumping up if she thought she heard anything untoward. Her parents became increasingly frustrated with her, having done their best to try to reassure her to no avail. They became even more concerned when Emmie started to reject all chewy or solid foods; she felt that she wouldn't be able to swallow these quickly and easily in case there was a noise. By the time they came to the clinic, Emmie was avoiding a large number of foods that she had previously quite happily eaten. Her diet had become very limited and her weight had dropped. She looked miserable and unhappy and her parents felt at a loss to know how to get her back to her old self.

Jake was 11 years old and had recently started secondary school. He was an active, friendly boy who had done well and been popular at his local primary school. He had found the much larger secondary school somewhat daunting, but by the start of his second term there, was beginning to feel more settled. Unfortunately, towards the end of January there was a small outbreak of mumps in the school and Jake was the youngest of the pupils to come down with it. Mumps is a notifiable disease and the school and local health care providers took the necessary action. Although Jake had had his vaccinations, it was explained to his parents that sometimes the second dose can fail, and a small number of people develop mumps despite being fully vaccinated. Jake had really been quite poorly with it and had experienced a lot of pain and discomfort when eating. He had missed quite a bit of school and when he returned, again felt quite overwhelmed by the size and unfamiliarity of the environment. He became much more subdued and developed increasing caution around what he would eat. He was clear that he felt some things might be too difficult to chew or hurt his throat and he didn't want to risk this as everything had been so horrible when he had mumps. When he attended clinic, Jake was restricted to eating well-cooked pasta and smooth soups. When these weren't available on the school lunch menu, he wasn't eating anything.

A brief word is perhaps in order here, about what is sometimes referred to as 'brand specificity'. This is when the person will only eat one particular brand of something: for example, they might only accept one brand of boxed oven fries and refuse other types of chips. They might restrict themselves to one flavour of one brand of yoghurt only, or in the case of a child with ARFID, they might become stuck on one brand of a particular baby food jar that they have never moved on from despite this no longer being at all age-appropriate. Many parents of children with ARFID will be familiar with this particular variant of brand loyalty, and even more familiar with the sense of dread should the manufacturer change the packaging. Even small changes in wording or appearance of the label or lid can result in refusal. Why is this? Is this driven by sensory preferences or it is driven by fear-based avoidance? It seems most likely that in many cases it is a combination of the two, and related to branded, mass-produced, packaged food being consistent and therefore predictable. The food of the preferred brand is likely to have become established as an acceptable taste and texture for the child with ARFID, but if the lid is now purple instead of green, or there is a different picture or different words on the packaging, they may sense a real risk that the content will be completely different. For most children with ARFID, that risk will simply not be worth taking and so the food will be refused. We will return to this issue of risk taking in later chapters (Chapter 5: What can I do? and Chapter 6: What is the best treatment for ARFID?) when we talk about *care*; what you can do to help with this and what treatments seem to work best.

You may have noticed that many of these aspects of eating behaviour, and the three common drivers of food choices discussed above (lack of interest; sensory characteristics of food; fear or concern about aversive consequences of eating), exist on a continuum. In other words, they may be present in all of us to a greater or lesser extent. It is not uncommon for our interest in food and eating to vary depending on our mood or level of pre-occupation with something. Sometimes our appetite does fluctuate for emotional reasons as well as due to the length of time since we last ate or topped up our energy levels. When very excited about something, some people find it harder to eat (whereas with others it can have the opposite effect). For example, if someone is engrossed in a book or in playing a computer game, a mealtime may come and go. Such fluctuations in interest in eating are normal. Most of us have likes and dislikes in terms of the taste, texture or smell of foods. We may all regard some foods as diffi-cult to eat, or disgusting, for one reason or another, and might be inclined to avoid them. Again, this is perfectly normal. And which of us hasn't approached food cautiously after a bout of vomiting, anxious to avoid a repeat of having to run to the bathroom? We can almost all recognise these three examples of drivers of the avoidance or restriction of food intake in ARFID, so how do we distinguish what is within the normal range and what is not? This is where the next part of the first requirement for a diagnosis of ARFID comes in.

Having established that there is avoidance or restriction of food intake (which may be the result of one or more of the contributing factors discussed above), the definition of ARFID additionally sets out that in turn, the limited intake must lead to one or more of four areas of impairment or interference with health, develop-ment or day-to-day functioning. This is important as one of the distinctions between normal variants of low interest in food, sen-sory preferences and concern around eating, and those present in ARFID, is that the latter have a significant negative impact. Let's look briefly at the areas highlighted in the formal definition of ARFID here, which we will revisit in more detail in the chapter on *consequences* (Chapter 4: What are the consequences of having ARFID?).

As mentioned, four areas of impact are listed, at least one of which must be present if a formal diagnosis is to be given. Firstly, there may be a failure to meet the individual's nutritional needs.

This means that the person with ARFID has such a restricted diet that they are missing key nutrients in their diet. If they have only been able to eat a limited range of foods for a while, they may develop significant nutritional deficiencies. That is, their body is not getting the vitamins and minerals (the micronutrients) or the full range of different types of food (the macronutrients, e.g. fat, carbohydrates, protein) that the human body requires. Inadequate nutrition associated with nutritional deficiencies is particularly concerning in children who are in a period of continuing development.

The second area of possible impact of the limited diet is that there may be a failure to meet the individual's energy (or calorie) needs. Here, the person with ARFID may struggle to manage sufficient amounts of food, or have a preference for foods which do not contain enough calories to sustain their needs. In children this can lead to failure to gain weight as expected, weight loss, and/or a slowing of their growth in terms of height. These are clear markers that intake is insufficient. Again we will discuss the impact of failure to meet energy needs in more detail later, when we consider *consequences* (in Chapter 4: What are the consequences of having ARFID?).

The third area of possible impact of the limited intake seen in ARFID, and listed in the definition, is that the person may be dependent on nutritional supplements taken by mouth, or dependent on tube feeding. Growing children should not, as a rule of thumb, be losing weight. They should also not be left with significant nutritional deficiencies that are likely to have an adverse effect on their health and development. When children do become very underweight or very nutritionally compromised, understandably, concern tends to rise. If there is a persistent difficulty in encouraging them to increase the amount or range of foods that they are eating, it may be suggested that prescribed nutritional supplements are used. These are usually given in two different ways: orally (via the mouth) or if that is not possible, via a tube into the stomach, or more rarely into part of the intestine called the jejunum. If a tube is used to facilitate dietary intake, this is known as 'enteral feeding'. When concerns arise, time frames in children are often much shorter than for adults; that is, they can get into difficulties with their weight and nutrition more quickly, as their fat and nutrient stores are generally proportionately smaller. Children also need adequate nutrition to ensure healthy development. For this reason, a number of children with long-standing avoidance and restriction behaviours may have their food intake supplemented with prescribed fortified drinks or powders or may be receiving some or the majority of their intake via a tube. If they are receiving supplements in this way, their weight, growth, and nutrition may be fine, but this does not mean they do not have a real difficulty with eating, which needs attention.

These three areas of impact discussed so far, considered toge-ther, mean that someone with ARFID could be underweight, but they could be in the appropriate weight range, or even above this, depending on their intake. If someone is limited to a very restric-ted but relatively high calorie diet, they may be nutritionally compromised but not necessarily underweight. In other words, just because a child is growing normally and their weight is not a concern, this does not necessarily mean that they do not have ARFID.

The fourth and final area of impact that may be related to the avoidant or restrictive intake, and included in the formal definition of ARFID, is impairment to 'psychosocial functioning'. This means that the individual's day-to-day functioning becomes com-promised in terms of their mental well-being and/or the ability to participate in normal social interactions. In other words, they may experience distress or difficulty in managing their emotional experience, and their relationships may be adversely affected. In children, impairment to psychological functioning can extend to interference with family functioning. This can arise as a direct consequence of the avoidance and restriction of food intake, as ARFID can have a negative impact on other members of the family as well. Again, we will look at this in more detail in our discussion of *consequences* (Chapter 4: What are the consequences of ARFID?).

At this point, we can summarise what ARFID is, in the form of Figure 1.1. Information relating to each circle is specified in the first requirement of the formal definition of ARFID, and needs to be obtained as part of the process of deciding if a diagnosis is

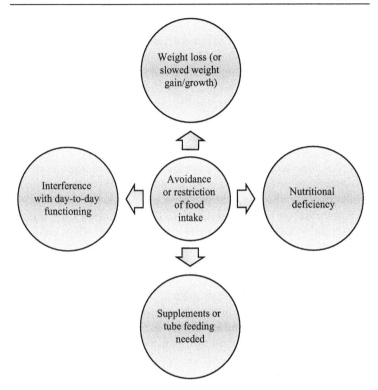

Figure 1.1 What ARFID is

appropriate. This first requirement essentially states that ARFID is characterised by avoidance or restriction of food intake, due to a range of possible underlying reasons (lack of interest; sensory-based; fear or concern about aversive consequences), which leads to at least one of the following four things: weight loss (or slowed weight gain or drop off in rate of growth in children); nutritional deficiency; dependence on supplements or tube feeds; interference with day-to-day functioning. In reality, the majority of children with ARFID will have one or more of these, with energy needs and/or nutritional needs typically not met.

We now need to turn our attention to the conditions that might mean we are *not* talking about ARFID: the exclusion criteria. In the formal definition of ARFID, the first of the three exclusion criteria states that the avoidance or restriction should not be due to lack of available food, or due to a practice that is considered culturally normal. For example, if a child has a very restricted diet because the family only has a very narrow range of things to eat in the home, we would not necessarily describe the child as having a feeding or eating difficulty. Similarly, if someone is avoiding foods as part of a religious observance, or other common practice in their community, this would not be considered a feeding or eating disorder. The second of the three exclusion considerations is that the avoidance or restriction of food intake does not stem primarily from concerns about weight or shape, such as is the case in anorexia nervosa or bulimia nervosa. If the main driver for limited intake is the desire to be thinner or to lose weight, then considering a diagnosis of anorexia or bulimia nervosa might be more appropriate. By definition, individuals with ARFID do not restrict their intake for these reasons. As we have seen, there are a range of other reasons behind the avoidance.

The third and final exclusion consideration is that the avoidance or restriction of food intake should not be better explained by another active medical condition that would make it difficult for anyone to eat. This might include, for example, a number of neurological problems which affect the ability to chew and swallow, or a gastrointestinal condition associated with severe food intolerances and malabsorption. In the presence of such conditions it may however still be possible for someone to develop ARFID; if their eating difficulties are over and above those that might be usually be expected under the circumstances and all the diagnostic criteria are met, then an additional diagnosis of ARFID may prove appropriate. It is often the case that children who have had a very difficult start in terms of their medical history, which has resulted in them needing assistance with their feeding, may be left with persistent eating difficulties long after there is any physical reason for this. Thus it is possible to develop ARFID in the context of other medical conditions, but these should not the main reason for the eating disturbance at the time ARFID may be being considered. Solly, who we have already met, is an example of this. He had a significant history of medical problems and related feeding difficulties earlier in life, but these persisted long after his physical health improved.

This final exclusion criterion also includes the requirement that the avoidance or restriction of food intake should not be better explained by another mental disorder. Perhaps the most straightforward examples are when someone has a significant, severe depression, or where the person is experiencing distressing delusional beliefs. We know that depression is often associated with appetite loss which can affect eating behaviour and cause weight loss. However, unlike in ARFID, appetite tends to pick up again with improvements in mood, with eating also returning to normal. Someone with a delusional belief, for example, that they are an animal, may only eat foods they think that animal should eat. Again, this change in eating behaviour is probably better explained by their impaired relationship with reality. As this improves, eating difficulties are likely to settle. A distinction is usually made between such examples of eating disturbance consistent with an acute episode of another mental disorder and ARFID. However, as with the consideration relating to medical conditions, it is possible that someone might develop ARFID in the context of another mental disorder. As long as all the diagnostic criteria for ARFID are met, and the eating difficulty is over and above what might be expected taking everything into account and requires treatment in its own right, then an additional diagnosis of ARFID may be warranted.

We can now add the exclusion considerations to our diagram, as in Figure 1.2. Taken together the circles represent what ARFID is – with one or more of the ring of four areas of impact required to be present – and the squares are the considerations or exclusion criteria that might mean this diagnosis is not appropriate.

We have now been through the formal definition of ARFID in some detail. These considerations allow the clinician to rule a diagnosis in, or rule it out. It may be helpful to understand two additional important aspects of the process of the clinician's decision as to whether a diagnosis is warranted, or not. The first relates to 'caseness' and the second to 'differential diagnoses'. Caseness is a term sometimes used to mean the extent to which diagnostic criteria apply to any one person. If some of the features of ARFID are present, but not all the required criteria have been

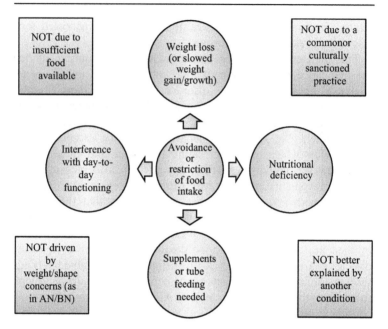

Figure 1.2 What ARFID is not

met, then the person will not receive a full diagnosis – they will not be a 'case' of ARFID. This language can seem very medical and impersonal and is often not used for this reason. It is quite off-putting to think of yourself as a case of this or that, when in reality whatever you are experiencing is an integral part of your experience. Nevertheless, it is current practice to draw a line around recognisable conditions in terms of their impact and severity. It is also important in being able to distinguish between difficulties that may be part of normal development, normal behavioural variations or normal emotional experience, and diffi- culties that require some additional input as they are related to significant impairment or distress.

Perhaps a good example here is what we know about young children's acceptance of vegetables. There is good research that shows that green vegetables are the least favourite foods amongst the majority of infants being weaned onto solids. Children inter-act with food with their senses and not uncommonly the bitter taste, characteristic of some green vegetables, is initially rejected. With repeated offering and encouragement, most children will gradually begin to widen their range of accepted foods. There is also good research to show that 'picky' or 'faddy' eating is very commonly reported by parents of pre-school children. If we think about this from a developmental perspective, this beha-viour makes sense at this stage of development. Toddlers and young children are beginning to assert their authority and start-ing to make their own choices about what they will and won't do. Children of this age have limited domains in which to express this. Most parents are familiar with the young child who is clearly demonstrating likes and dislikes when it comes to food, and who may refuse or reject certain foods in quite forceful ways! Research shows that, over time, this earlier pickiness tends to reduce, with the majority of children beginning to eat or accept broader diets by the age of five or six years. Young children with ARFID will differ from children displaying this more normal pattern, in terms of the severity of the impact of their limited intake. It is very unusual for developmentally normal picky eating in toddlers to result in weight loss or failure to gain weight over a prolonged period, or for their growth to falter as a con-sequence of picky intake. These are not the children who require prescribed nutritional supplements from the doctor or a dietitian, to ensure they are able to thrive. It can be hard for parents to make these distinctions, because they may be understandably concerned about refusal behaviour and limited acceptance of different foods. On the other hand, we know that making the distinction between normal pickiness and ARFID in a younger child can also be difficult for some clinicians. Children with ARFID are likely to be struggling in terms of their eating beha-viour and interactions to a significant extent, whereas more normal faddiness does not have the same impact. A considera-tion of caseness is therefore part of the process of deciding if someone meets diagnostic criteria.

The other main area that needs to be considered, is whether there might be something else entirely that is accounting for the difficulties. This process is known as considering differential diagnoses. A number of conditions might initially look similar in terms of reported or observed features, and part of arriving at a diagnosis is to make sure the most relevant ones have been considered and the correct diagnosis is made. We know from the above, that such considerations form one of the exclusion criteria for ARFID; if there is a better explanation for the avoidance or restriction of food intake, a diagnosis of ARFID may not be appropriate. The most obvious differential diagnosis in children from around the age of eight years and up who have significantly restricted eating behaviour is perhaps anorexia nervosa. Anorexia nervosa and ARFID share the characteristic of limited eating, but there are number of key differences. Some of the main ones that may be encountered are highlighted in Table 1.1.

Table 1.1 Points of possible similarity and difference between ARFID and anorexia nervosa

Similarities	Differences
Weight loss (NB in a subset of ARFID only)	Weight/shape issues driving the restriction (in AN not ARFID)
Limited intake	Behaviours that are intended to promote weight loss (in AN not ARFID)
Impact on family life and arrangements around eating with mealtime arguments and stress	Onset of difficulty (can be very early in ARFID)
Social isolation – struggles to eat with others or when out	Prior eating behaviour (often unproblematic before AN; in ARFID more often longstanding)
Affects family members (e.g. anxiety/ low mood/anger/frustration)	Composition of diet (tends to be low calorie in AN due to wish to control weight)
The individual may not be motivated to change their eating or recognise the extent of its impact	Role of self-evaluation (in AN self-worth tends to be judged in terms of weight and shape)

There are of course other conditions that might mimic some of the features of ARFID as we have seen, such as gastrointestinal conditions, difficulties that affect oral-motor functioning, and depression. When conducting an assessment, most clinicians will ask lots of questions about things other than what your child is eating for this reason. They will be running through the requirements of a range of other conditions in their mind, to be certain they are not giving a wrong diagnosis.

Having been through the formal definition of ARFID as it currently stands, and considered the issues of caseness and differential diagnosis, there are two more aspects of the 'What is ARFID?' question that might be helpful to set out in a bit more detail before we finish this *characterisation* chapter. The first relates to the question of whether there are clear sub-types of ARFID, and the second to the question of whether ARFID should be considered a feeding disorder or whether it is better thought of as an eating disorder (and indeed whether this matters!).

There is currently quite a lot of discussion about whether there are clear sub-types of ARFID. We know from how ARFID has been defined, that a number of the more commonly occurring reasons behind the avoidance or restriction of food intake have been included in its description. These three, now hopefully familiar, examples – lack of interest, sensory based avoidance, and restriction or avoidance based on concern about unwanted consequences – are not always mutually exclusive. Hallie's eating pattern illustrates this.

Hallie came to the clinic with her parents, who described longstanding feeding difficulties, dating back to weaning. Hallie had initially been a hungry baby, who seemed to enjoy her milk feeds. Initially, she transitioned well onto purees and smooth foods, including blended family meals. Her parents described not really having many concerns about her intake until she was between 12 and 18 months of age, although they had begun to notice that she was not keen on finger foods and seemed to be stuck on foods of a smooth consistency. They had managed to achieve some successes with a few more solid foods over the subsequent years, but at the age of four and a half and due to start school in a few months, Hallie was still struggling to accept anything approaching an age-appropriate range of foods. Her parents expressed concern that she would not be able to cope with lunchtime at school as she was still reliant on having most of her foods blended. To make matters worse, she had spent a weekend with her grandparents a few weeks previously, while her parents attended a wedding. Hallie had a cold at the time and had been reluctant to see them go. Her grandmother had mashed rather than blended her food, so that it was much lumpier than Hallie was used to. During her first meal Hallie had gagged on the feel of the food in her mouth and became upset as her grandmother had insisted she should keep eating. She ended up crying so much that she vomited at the table. On return home, Hallie had insisted that she couldn't have anything with lumps in as she would be sick, reverting to smoothly blended foods only and dropping some of the more solid foods her parents had worked hard to introduce.

In Hallie's case therefore, at the time she came to the clinic, food avoidance was driven both by sensory-based avoidance and by a fear of being sick. We also know from looking at data sets from clinics seeing large numbers of children with such difficulties, that there may be more than one driver of the avoidance or restriction of food intake. It may be that one reason is more dominant, or they may be equally dominant. In addition, there may be completely different reasons underlying the avoidance or restriction which may accompany one or more of the three examples we are now familiar with, or they may be present without any of these three more commonly occurring reasons. In this way it can be helpful to think of ARFID as an 'umbrella diagnosis'; it includes types and patterns of eating behaviour that may differ between one person and the next. The five children already described – Solly, Kai, Emmie, Jake and Hallie – all had ARFID, but all are slightly different.

In order to definitively determine the answer to the question of whether there are distinct subtypes of ARFID, we need more data. We need to know the answer to lots of sub-questions: do different types of ARFID presentation respond differently to specific treatment approaches?; are certain variants of ARFID always associated with specific other features? (which we will discuss further in Chapter 2: Who can develop ARFID?, when we discuss *correlates*); do some types of ARFID run in families?; and many more such questions.

One area of interest in this respect is the eating pattern referred to by some as 'orthorexia'. This word comes from the Greek prefix 'ortho-' which means straight, correct, upright – as in orthodontist, someone who specialises in straightening teeth; and the Greek suffix '-orexis', which means desire, or appetite – as in anorexia, where 'an-' means absence of, so that an-orexia means absence of appetite. Orthorexia has been defined in a number of different ways and is not currently a formal diagnosis. It is often described as an extreme pre-occupation or obsession with eating food that is considered to be healthy, or a condition characterised by the person taking extreme care to cut out all foods that they consider potentially harmful. It can be argued that it is possible to include orthorexia under the ARFID umbrella, where the avoidance or restriction of food intake is linked to an extreme concern about aversive or unwanted consequences of eating certain foods, leading to inadequate intake. Could it be that orthorexia might be recognised as a sub-type of ARFID, as long as all the other criteria are met? At present we do not have solid answers to these questions relating to possible sub-types, but there has certainly been a rise in research looking into such issues. For now therefore, we are in the position of there being insufficient evidence to determine whether it will be possible to delineate distinct sub-types of ARFID. As ever, that picture may change as understanding improves.

Finally, is ARFID a feeding disorder or an eating disorder? What is the difference between feeding and eating? We often use the term 'feeding' in relation to those who are dependent on another person for their nutritional intake. This might include babies, young children, people with a physical disability, or the very frail or elderly. Feeding somehow denotes an element of dependent interaction, with the person being fed receiving the food from another. However, if we are reading a newspaper article about the challenges of 'feeding soldiers in a warzone' we are certainly not going to imagine that this is about each soldier being fed by another person. Feeding in this context means providing food for. Eating usually has more active or volitional connotations, with the action of eating being engaged in by the individual concerned. However, in everyday language we use these terms quite loosely and interchangeably; 'What am I going to feed the children?' and 'What am I going to give the children to eat?' are similar in meaning. Formal definitions of feeding and eating reflect these differences, with the verb 'to feed' meaning to give someone or something food or drink to eat, to nourish or to nurture. The verb 'to eat' is usually defined as the act of consuming food (or other substances) through putting in the mouth and chewing and swallowing.

The terms 'feeding disorder' and 'eating disorder' are therefore somewhat confusing. When many people hear 'eating disorder' they think of anorexia nervosa or bulimia nervosa. 'Feeding disorder' tends to be a term associated with the very young or those who are less able physically or developmentally. ARFID is referred to as a feeding disorder by some but described as an eating disorder by others. So which is correct? We have already seen that ARFID was introduced into the diagnostic classification system as a replacement and extension of feeding disorder of infancy or early childhood. However, ARFID is certainly characterised by eating difficulties in the form of avoidance or restriction. We have also seen that it can apply to children, adolescents, and adults, and now sits in a section called Feeding and Eating Disorders. Some people clearly feel very strongly about this issue, but ultimately whether we think of ARFID as a feeding disorder or an eating disorder should not make any difference to our collective responsibility to recognise it, and to manage and treat it to the best of our ability. We will return to some of the challenges posed by this confusion in use of terms when we move to the discussion about *care* (Chapter 6: What is the best treatment for ARFID?).

Some readers may have noticed something that might at first glance appear to be a typing error. When discussing the fourth version of the DSM system, reference has been made to DSM-IV.

However, when discussing the fifth version of the system (the one that contains ARFID as a diagnosis), DSM-5 has been used. This change from Roman numerals to Arabic, or conventional, numbers is intentional and has been made for a very important reason. Diagnostic categories are not set in stone; in relation to mental health they represent what is deemed to be the best way to capture a recognisable pattern, or patterns, of behaviour, beliefs, and emotional experiences that are associated with distress or impairment, at any one time. It is not possible to provide the last word on the answer to the question addressed in this chapter: 'What is ARFID?' The way we describe and define things is based on evidence. What we know about ARFID and how it has been defined so far, is based on careful scrutiny of all relevant available evidence. The evidence that we have access to is constantly changing as research is carried out, as we listen to those affected and document what they are telling us, and as clinicians gain experience in treating people with ARFID. The final wording for the description of ARFID in ICD-11 is expected to be endorsed in 2019, with the majority of the world's countries reporting on its presence from 2022. It is not yet known if these developments will result in changes to our conceptualisation of ARFID as a form of feeding or eating disorder. In light of this, the switch to Arabic numerals seems appropriate; the intention being that if and when compelling evidence clearly points to necessary changes, modifications can be made to definitions in line with this new knowledge, and criteria updated to version 5.1, version 5.2 and so on. It may well be that in 5 or 10 years' time, there will be some differences in how the question at the heart of this chapter – the question of what ARFID is – should be answered. However, for now the discussion above represents agreed and accepted views and we will proceed with this in mind.

Chapter 2

Who can develop ARFID?

This chapter will cover what we know about the epidemiology of ARFID, that is, what we know about its distribution in the population. This will address the 'Who can develop ARFID?' question. We will look at the further detail of this by considering whether there are specific risk factors and by noticing common co-occurring characteristics and conditions. This chapter is the *correlates* chapter, discussing things that are 'co-related' or have been observed to be present alongside ARFID.

An important aspect of the 'Who can develop ARFID?' question is the consideration of whether there are any factors that place one person more at risk of developing ARFID than another. As with almost all other areas relating to ARFID, research on such risk factors remains limited. The identification of risk factors relies on the ability to track back and discover whether there are individual characteristics, patterns of events or situations that might predispose one person more than another to developing a certain condition. Better still is tracking forward, that is, following a group of people carefully to see whether certain characteristics measured at an earlier point in time might predict greater likelihood of developing a condition. This type of forward tracking generally produces more reliable and better quality information. Tracking back is often less satisfactory as there may be missing information, or some things that now appear useful to know which were not documented at the time.

It is usual in health research to try to identify risk factors, as this can assist with preventative efforts. A well-known example is cigarette smoking, which we now know is a major risk factor for lung cancer. This was first identified in the 1950s and since then research findings accumulated, demonstrating a clear link between smoking and increased risk of lung cancer. As awareness of this grew over the subsequent decades, so too did anti-smoking public health campaigns. These campaigns were designed to inform people about the risks of smoking and to encourage them to change their behaviour. This has achieved some success with smoking, with far fewer people smoking cigarettes now compared to 50 or even 20 years ago and deaths from lung cancer dropping, particularly in men. Through targeting and reducing risk factors, in this case smoking behaviour, it can be possible to reduce the number of people who develop a condition.

This is all well and good in the case of 'modifiable' risk factors, that is, things that can in theory be changed. However, not all risk factors are to do with behaviour, which can potentially be altered; some are to do with age, sex, family background or race. Many such genetic or physical characteristics are not possible to change and so are known as 'non-modifiable' risk factors. For example, having a relative with early onset heart disease may mean you have a higher risk of developing heart disease yourself, than someone with no family history of heart disease. However, you can make sure you exercise and eat sensibly to moderate this risk. Here, the familial susceptibility is the non-modifiable risk factor, and diet and exercise are the modifiable risk factors. If you are from an Afro-Caribbean background, you have a higher risk of having sickle-cell disease than someone from a European background. In this example, the genetic trait for sickle cell disease is found more commonly in people originating from specific parts of the world, including Africa, the Caribbean, the Middle East and parts of Asia. In the case of non-modifiable risk factors, the usual approach is to try to increase vigilance of those most at risk and identification of early signs and symptoms of the condition of interest. This is often achieved through screening or monitoring programmes and initiatives. The aim of these is to reduce the overall risks to the individual through early identification and early treatment. Understanding which risk factors are linked with specific conditions is important in terms of the health of the population. They can help us a great deal in predicting who might develop a condition and in our attempts to prevent ill-health and disease.

In relation to ARFID, it seems probable that, as with most conditions, we are dealing with a range of both modifiable and non-modifiable risk factors. We know that different people have slightly different forms of ARFID, with some degree of variation in which features are most prominent. However, we do not yet have years' worth of research to help us be sure about patterns relating to the onset of ARFID. In particular, we do not have information from the more robust forward tracking studies to allow us to reliably conclude that characteristic A, B or C is likely to increase the likelihood of developing ARFID. However, we do have a growing number of observations about things that appear to go hand in hand with ARFID in some individuals. Slowly, patterns of these correlates are beginning to emerge. Correlates and risk factors are often linked and so it is worth spending some time on these here.

A number of studies have been carried out looking at groups of older children and adolescents seen in clinics and in-patient settings for treatment of an eating disorder. These have generally been places specialising in the treatment of anorexia nervosa and bulimia nervosa. A fairly consistent picture has been reported, that generally between 10 and 30% of young people seen in such settings have ARFID. Furthermore, as a group, those with ARFID tend to be slightly younger than those with anorexia nervosa and bulimia nervosa, and to have experienced eating difficulties for much longer before they are seen in these clinics. These things are to do with the *course* of ARFID which we will return to later (Chapter 7: What about the future?).

Have there been any correlates identified through these studies that could be risk factors? Let's consider the usual non-modifiable risk factors first. In relation to age, these studies can't tell us very much about age as a risk factor as they are focussed on what might turn out to be a small section of the population of people who develop ARFID. Most of these studies include individuals aged between eight and 18 years, but we know that ARFID certainly occurs in younger children and also that it occurs in adults.

Based on clinical observation and the existing published literature, difficulties resembling ARFID have been most commonly described in children in the two to 12 year age range. However, this requires whole population studies to be able to determine if this is indeed the age range we might consider to be linked to the greatest risk. Aside from commenting that some children and young people with ARFID are being seen in these particular treatment programmes at a slightly younger age than those with anorexia nervosa, the studies are unable to tell us a great deal. Our current knowledge about earliest age of onset of anorexia nervosa suggests that this is around seven or eight years of age, whereas we know that ARFID can be present much sooner. The findings from these studies therefore make sense in terms of what we know about of age of onset.

Turning to sex, these studies of young people in eating disorder clinics and in-patient settings show a higher percentage of boys in the group with ARFID, compared to those with anorexia nervosa and bulimia nervosa. This too, is difficult to interpret on the basis of these studies alone, as they almost certainly do not include a group of young people with ARFID that is representative of everyone who meets diagnostic criteria. It does seem quite likely though, that there may be more boys with ARFID than boys with anorexia nervosa. ARFID is not driven by weight or shape concerns which have long had a greater, although not exclusive, association with being female, whereas many of the drivers for avoidance and restriction in ARFID are perhaps less gender specific.

In relation to familial risk, or risk related to racial background, and any clear correlates in these domains, so far these studies looking at differences specifically between young people with ARFID and those with anorexia nervosa and bulimia nervosa tell us little. However, they do suggest that those with ARFID tend to also have much higher rates of anxiety related difficulties as well as other conditions, including attention deficit hyperactivity disorder (ADHD) and a range of medical conditions. We are going to concentrate on *causes* and possible causal pathways in our next chapter (Chapter 3: Why does someone develop ARFID?) and will be exploring some of the ways in which anxiety, attention difficulties and medical difficulties might contribute more directly to the development of ARFID there.

What else do we know about *correlates* of ARFID? Another group of individuals that has been identified as having higher rates of avoidant and restrictive eating behaviours are children and young people with autism spectrum disorder (ASD). This is a term that captures a number of different presentations, including what used to be known as Asperger's syndrome, also sometimes known as 'high functioning' autism. People with autism vary a great deal in terms of their skills and abilities. As the term autism spectrum disorder suggests, a range of difficulties can be present, and many traits associated with autism are found to a lesser extent in people who do not meet diagnostic criteria. The key features of autism include difficulties with communicating and interacting with others, a tendency to engage in repetitive patterns of certain behaviours, having narrow interests, and a different response to sensory stimulation than most other people. Autism can be accompanied by intellectual difficulties; in fact these two things co-occur frequently. However, autism can go hand in hand with average or very high levels of intellectual ability. It can be accompanied by language impairment, although again this is not always the case and some people with autism have age-appropriate or very high language skills. Autism is often referred to as a 'neurodevelopmental' condition, which essentially means that it is present from an early age. In some people, difficulties may take a long time to become apparent or have an impact. Most people are recognised as having autism in childhood, but in some, it may not be until adolescence or even adulthood that their difficulties have a major effect. As with most conditions, having a diagnosis of autism is linked with the person experiencing significant difficulties in day-to-day functioning. Again, we will explore the shared aspects of autism and ARFID, in particular the tendency to stick to routines or the same behaviours, and the increased sensitivity to sensory input in the *causes* chapter next (Chapter 3: Why does someone develop ARFID?).

Staying with the discussion about neurodevelopmental conditions, this cluster of presentations also includes children with intellectual developmental difficulties which can result in delays in terms of the child's learning and in delays in acquiring the same skills and abilities as their peers. Sometimes young children are referred to as having 'global developmental delay', a term that can be used when the usual milestones are not met. Such children often experience difficulties with feeding and eating. Sometimes this may be a question of development alone, that is, the child is delayed in their feeding development as well as in all other aspects of their development. However, some children with intellectual developmental difficulties do have significant eating problems which meet the diagnostic criteria for ARFID and need additional attention.

The other neurodevelopmental condition to mention here, which we know can co-occur with ARFID in a number of children, is attention deficit hyperactivity disorder, or ADHD. We have already seen above that this association has been identified as occurring more commonly in the comparisons between young people over the age of eight years with ARFID and those with anorexia nervosa. ADHD is also seen in younger children who experience clear difficulties with focus, concentration, and attention. An added complication with children with ADHD in relation to eating is the fact that they may have been prescribed medication for this condition. The most commonly prescribed medications are known as stimulants. You might think a stimulant is the last thing a child who can't sit still needs, but what these drugs are doing is stimulating the part of the brain that helps them pay attention and manage their behaviour. One of the well-known side effects of these drugs is that they often cause a loss of appetite. Medication related loss of appetite resulting in reduced intake does not mean a child should also be described as having ARFID if this is the direct and only cause of the restriction. However, if your child has ADHD and really struggles with their eating irrespective of whether they are on medication or not, they may well meet diagnostic criteria for ARFID as well. It is often the case that many parents express concern about starting their children on ADHD medication if their child is already struggling to eat enough due to the worry that they may lose even more weight. However, in many instances, the medicine can actually help them also focus on eating and so this does not occur. We will return to this in the chapter on *care* (Chapter 6: What is the best treatment for ARFID?).

In this relatively brief chapter, we have considered the question 'Who can develop ARFID?' We can conclude that people of any age can have ARFID; this is well documented and well recognised. In terms of the lower age range, in theory there is no lower age limit, however, in practice certain considerations seem appropriate. As we have seen, ARFID is classified as a mental disorder. 'Mental' takes its origin from the Latin for in or of the mind. Mental disorders are related to behaviour, emotions, thoughts, beliefs, and attitudes, i.e. things going on in the brain that are significantly different to the experiences of other people and importantly cause impairment or distress to the individual involved. It can be difficult to think of an infant with feeding difficulties as having a formal mental disorder. We can't readily determine an infant's thoughts, beliefs and attitudes. We can observe their facial expressions and listen to their babble and noises and only infer how they might be feeling from this. Infants also have limited ability to exert control over their own behaviour. Self-regulation is generally thought to start at around one year of age, and as every parent knows, usually develops quickly thereafter. However, until the age of two or so, there is significant variability in this. For these reasons, it seems appropriate to avoid giving a diagnosis of ARFID in very young children below the age of two years. By this time, feeding development has usually progressed to a stage where difficulties related to the child's behaviour, thoughts and feelings, if they exist, will be clearly apparent.

In addition, we know that between the ages of two and five years or so, many children engage in picky eating. Research involving large groups of children shows that in the majority this type of eating behaviour is not so severe that it affects their health, growth or development. It also shows that the majority of children tend to broaden their diets as time goes by. This does not mean to say that all picky eating should be dismissed as nothing to worry about, because we also know that children with a very high degree of pickiness and those in whom the tendency to be very selective persists, appear to be more likely to have or to develop ARFID. Thus in terms of the youngest age a diagnosis of ARFID might be appropriate, it is possible to put forward the argument that this should be two years. However, this is at present a matter of discussion and different clinicians might adopt different practices.

In conclusion therefore, we should probably assume that many different types of people can develop ARFID. We shouldn't dismiss anyone as not being the type to develop ARFID nor should we necessarily assume that anyone with the correlates we have discussed in this chapter (e.g. anxiety, ASD, ADHD) is going to have difficulties in relation to the avoidance or restriction of food intake. We simply do not know enough at this stage to be more specific.

Chapter 3

Why does someone develop ARFID?

We have established that both boys and girls (and men and women) can have ARFID, and that we would use this term as long as diagnostic criteria are met in anyone over the age of two years. In the previous chapter's discussion of *correlates* (Chapter 2: Who can develop ARFID?), we have also seen that ARFID is often associated with certain other conditions. In particular, anxiety, autism, ADHD, developmental delay, and a range of medical conditions have been noted to co-occur at slightly higher rates than we might otherwise expect. We have also recognised that none of these other conditions need to be present and that someone can develop ARFID in the absence of any other type of difficulty. We are now moving on to the question of why this might happen; why does a person develop ARFID? This chapter provides a summary of what we know about *causes*.

It is probably worth stating clearly that there is unlikely to be one single cause of ARFID. We know from reviewing its *characteristics* (Chapter 1: What is ARFID?) that this is an umbrella term; ARFID includes a range of different variants of eating disturbance, all having avoidance or restriction of food intake as a shared feature. It does not seem unreasonable to conclude that these different expressions may result from different possible pathways. We undoubtedly have a long way to go to determine on the basis of research evidence exactly which pathways or combinations of events or conditions lead to ARFID.

Does the absence of certainty about what has caused a problem matter? If you are like many other parents and carers, you may be left wondering why your child doesn't eat like other children. What could you have done or not done to avoid being in the situation you are now in? We know from discussions with caregivers that this 'why?' question is one that keeps people awake at night. It can be the cause of arguments when one person's version of what has caused the child to avoid or restrict foods is very different to another's. It can lead to inconsistent attempts to set things right, which can be confusing and is unlikely to be helpful for the child. It can lead to feelings of guilt or blame, emotions which are rarely of help to anyone concerned. It can result in resentment between parents, and in some cases multiple strongly held views about why a child has ARFID can contribute to stress, unhappiness, and become a whole separate issue in their own right. Clearly this is the last thing any family needs when they are trying to ensure their child eats enough.

How then do we reconcile this lack of certainty about the cause of the difficulty with being able to find a way to answer the 'why' question? One simple way to try to do this is illustrated in the diagram in Figure 3.1. This is a deceptively minimalist representation and an

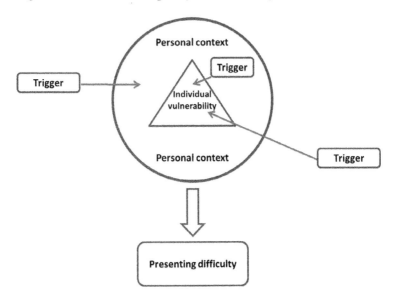

Figure 3.1 Model for understanding the development of difficulties

example of a more complex 'biopsychosocial' model for understanding the development of difficulties. The biopsychosocial
approach to understanding health and illness was first put forward by
an American doctor called George Engel in 1977 (see Engel 1980,
1997) and has since become widely adopted. Essentially this approach
proposes that health and illness result from the interplay of biological
factors, psychological factors and social factors. This seems to make
good sense and this approach has been shown to be helpful in understanding the development of a whole range of conditions, including
chronic pain, heart disease and depression. It can also be helpful in
understanding why someone might develop ARFID. Take a look at
Figure 3.1 and we will go over the elements in more detail.

In the centre you will see a triangle with 'individual vulnerability'. Each of us is more or less vulnerable to developing a
whole range of conditions. In part this is determined by our family
history and our temperament, both of which are related to our
genetic makeup. In part it is determined by our own development,
and by our personal and medical history. In part our vulnerability
can be raised or lowered through our actions, behaviours, and
lifestyle choices. Any or all of these things can mean that one
person is more vulnerable to developing a certain condition than
another. As individuals, none of us lives in total isolation; we all
live in a context. The circle is labelled 'personal context' to capture this. The extent to which our individual vulnerability to
develop something is expressed often depends on our interaction
with our environment. Our environment includes our family and
our interactions with family members as well as our wider social
networks such as friends, school, university, and work. It includes
our religious and cultural communities, as well as our social
backgrounds in terms of poverty or wealth. We pick up different
habits, form different attitudes, adopt certain lifestyles, or are
constrained in these respects, through influences and input from
our own personal context. For each of us, as with individual vulnerability, our personal context is unique. Finally, there are a
number of rectangles containing the word 'trigger'. These represent events that can tip us into having a particular condition
(represented here by 'presenting difficulty'). Triggers are sometimes
mistakenly understood as *causes*. They are perhaps better thought of

as part of a wider picture of contributing factors. These triggers can be things we do ourselves (the one within the individual vulnerability box); things that occur in our personal context, which have an effect on us (the trigger within the circle); or things that happen in wider society. Let's run through a quick example. If your child is born with a vulnerability to develop asthma, this may or may not be expressed depending on the air quality of where they live, or if anyone in the family smokes. A trigger may be the child catching a cold or as an adolescent taking up smoking. The development of the asthma is 'caused' by an interplay of different factors. We will return to this way of thinking about *causes* of ARFID having reviewed what we know can be contributing factors.

Let's start with the three most commonly identified drivers of the avoidance or restriction of food intake: low interest in food or eating; avoidance based on sensory aspects of food or eating; and avoidance related to concern about possible negative consequences of eating. We will unpick each of these in turn to try to understand what might have contributed to them and what might be maintaining them, thereby causing the difficulties you may be seeing in your own child, or another individual with ARFID.

Low interest in food or eating

Interest in food and eating is a more complicated matter than you might think! It includes a number of components, including the availability of food, whether you are hungry, and the extent to which you 'fancy' different foods. Low interest in food or eating can therefore stem from a number of different things with a number of possible pathways that may be relevant to explore. For the purposes of our consideration of low interest in food and eating in the context of ARFID it can be useful to consider those related to poor hunger recognition as well as those related to not really 'fancying' food, which is sometimes known as low 'avidity', or a lack of eagerness or enthusiasm to eat. We also need to consider other reasons which might be associated with low interest in food and eating, for example, when eating requires a lot of effort or when we are unwell. Some of these reasons are captured in Figure 3.2 and are discussed in more detail below.

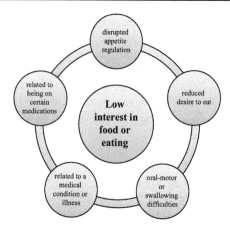

Figure 3.2 Possible causes of low interest in food or eating

Disrupted appetite regulation

Most infants are naturally quite efficient when it comes to self-regulation around feeding. They tend to cry and feed when they are hungry and are less interested when they are not. There can of course be individual differences in appetite right from the start, with some babies being described as hungry babies whereas others may give cues that they are hungry less often or take less during feeds. In normal feeding development, children adapt their intake according to their energy needs, relying on the presence of a caregiver able to respond to their cues to do so. It is extraordinary that this process of the baby crying or signalling hunger in other ways, with the mother responding by feeding, occurs so often without undue difficulty. Over time this gradually settles into a rhythm that meets the child's needs.

There are however, a number of factors that can interrupt this process. Reema's story is one example.

Reema is her parents' third child. She has two older sisters, each of the three girls separated by around 18 months in age, and one younger brother, two years younger than Reema.

Reema's mother had a difficult pregnancy when carrying her. She suffered from sickness throughout and became unwell herself with a number of chest infections. Reema subsequently had a lengthy and difficult birth and both mother and baby appeared exhausted. Reema struggled to feed adequately as she tended to fall asleep or give up sucking after a short while. Despite attempts to increase her intake through frequent feeds and trying her on a bottle as well as the breast, her weight fell below a safe threshold. The doctor explained to Reema's parents that a feeding tube was needed to ensure that Reema received enough nutrition. This would be in the form of nasogastric tube feeds; the hospital team recommended that Reema should be given a specially formulated feed for infants via a tube going from her nose down to her stomach. Once adequate nutrition and weight gain had been established, the plan would be to recommence feeding via the breast or bottle. The doctor explained that babies generally managed this much better after they had had a 'top-up'.

In Reema's case, however, things were not so straightforward. Each time they tried to introduce a bottle while she still had the tube in place, she became distressed and refused to feed. They considered what best to do together with the team looking after her. The possibility was suggested that she might be uncomfortable with the tube in place as well as a teat in her mouth and that this might be putting her off. A decision was made to remove the tube and to try to offer the bottle without anything else around her nose and mouth. Reema's parents were advised to keep trying for the next 24 hours and to let the team know how they got on. Over the next few days, Reema steadfastly refused to accept the bottle. Her parents struggled to get anything other than a small amount of fluid into her. Once again mother and baby became exhausted and the decision was made to replace the tube. Reema settled again onto the tube feeds, which she seemed to accept without difficulty.

This pattern was repeated on a few occasions until Reema was about six months old. The hospital's guidelines were that children should generally not have a nasogastric tube in place for longer than three months. If there was agreement that a child continued to need tube feeding, then the usual practice would be to discuss the possibility of placing a gastrostomy tube allowing the child to be fed directly into the stomach. The doctor discussed this with Reema's parents and explained that sometimes it can be easier to try to introduce food and drink by mouth with a gastrostomy in place. Although Reema's parents were not happy with the prospect of Reema having surgery to put the tube in, they could see that she was not yet willing to take enough by mouth to be able to manage without despite repeated attempts to achieve this.

Reema eventually moved to gastrostomy feeds around the age of nine months. She and her parents settled into a routine of tube feeds which she tolerated well. The medical team were happy with Reema's growth and development and advised her parents to keep trying her with food and drink. They did this, but Reema rarely seemed interested and did not appear to enjoy anything they offered to her. When they tried to reduce the amount of feed they put down the tube, Reema did not seem to feel hungrier and never asked for food.

When Reema came to the clinic at the age of five years, she still had the gastrostomy in place and relied on tube feeds for just over half of her total intake. Each time they had tried to cut the amount of feed, she would struggle to gain weight and a few times lost weight so they had to increase the feed to more than she had been on previously. When seen for assessment, Reema was well. She would eat small amounts of food with the family, but not enough to meet her needs and almost always without enthusiasm. Her mother could not recall her ever having asked for food.

Reema had never had the opportunity to learn to self-regulate as she had been tube-fed almost all her life. She had a very poor awareness of when she was hungry, possibly because she had never had to depend on signalling hunger to be fed. Sometimes there is a clear, ongoing medical reason why children need to be tube-fed for a long time, but in Reema's case none had been identified. She had early faltering growth and subsequent tube feeding –

necessary at the time – had appeared to disrupt her appetite regulation. In the absence of any current medical explanation to explain her restricted intake, with a dependence on tube feeding that was no longer considered medically necessary and clear low interest in food and eating, Reema was given a diagnosis of ARFID. We will return to how children like Reema can be supported to eat in the section on *care* (Chapter 6: What is the best treatment for ARFID?).

Whilst prolonged tube feeding can disrupt the development of normal appetite regulation, it does not always have this effect. When tube feeding is required because of an underlying medical condition it is most commonly the case that once the medical condition has been addressed, most children will transition on to, or back to, oral feeding.

Reduced desire to eat

Most of us are familiar with some degree of variation in our desire to eat certain foods or to eat more generally. We might think 'I really fancy an omelette' one day, or 'I don't really feel like fish tonight' another. We might come back from shopping thinking 'I really need my lunch', or sit down to a meal saying 'I don't feel quite ready for dinner'. This variation is completely normal and not always simply to do with whether we are hungry or not. However, it is generally temporary, so that we don't end up eating omelettes at every meal, or never eating much dinner because we are never quite ready. In contrast, in people with ARFID a reduced desire to eat may be present to an extreme degree which does not readily self-correct in a short period of time. So why might that be? There are three factors in particular, that may play a role in contributing to the reduced desire to eat often seen in ARFID: mood; arousal; and habitual undereating.

Mood

As with many aspects of ARFID, this one also occurs on a spectrum that we can almost all recognise. If we are feeling a strong emotion, negative or positive, this can affect our eating behaviour.

Some of us will have a tendency to eat more than we normally might and some less. Imagine someone who is excited that a friend or relative they haven't seen for a long time is coming to visit. Everything is prepared and the only thing left to do is wait till the expected time of arrival. Some of us will pace around, finding it hard to settle, making sure everything is ready, feeling mounting excitement but absolutely no desire to eat anything. Others will feel equally excited but find they keep going back to the biscuit tin. In this way, a positive emotion, such as excitement, can increase or reduce our usual desire to eat. Another example that many will recognise is related to a negative emotion: feeling very sad. For some, feeling miserable is associated with eating a greater amount than usual. For others, unhappiness is associated with picking at food and failing to eat anything other than a small amount. Experiencing grief is another example; many people will lose some interest in eating after the death of someone they love. In this way strong positive and negative emotions can affect eating in many of us. Assuming we are not depressed or there is another clear reason to explain this increase or decrease in desire to eat, this tends to self-correct. However, in ARFID the effect that emotional experience can have on reducing eating behaviour tends to be persistent and more extreme.

Children with ARFID may be struggling with their mood. Some may be prone to crying at the slightest thing and can wear everyone down with attempts to avoid upsets. Others seem constantly nervous and on edge. We have seen that people with ARFID often have co-occurring difficulties with anxiety. In children, this might not be at the level of a formal diagnosis, but more a character trait. Some children are worriers; they may be cautious and timid in all aspects of their behaviour. Other children seem to be angry or frustrated all the time; nothing is quite right. Some may seem quite flat and don't appear to have much desire to do anything very much.

Learning to manage emotional experience is part of normal development, but for some children this will be much harder than others. We know that individual characteristics related to emotional processing run in families. Thinking back to the diagram in Figure 3.1, we can think of these aspects as components of the individual's vulnerability. Children's temperaments differ; one child will be more or less prone to be anxious than another. Given that emotional experience, or mood, can reduce the desire to eat, it is certainly worth considering as a possible contributing factor to a child's food avoidance or restricted intake.

Arousal

Arousal is a word that is thought to originate from terms meaning awake or arise. It is perhaps most often used in everyday language in association with sexual attraction, but its meaning is much broader. In general, the state of being aroused is akin to being alert, ready to go, or stimulated. Over-arousal or over-stimulation is generally not a good thing. Common examples are the adolescent who has been playing on the computer too long and too close to bedtime; the adult who is so busy and stressed at work that lying in bed making mental to-do lists displaces sleep; the child who has had so much fun with their friend that they behave very badly when it comes to picking-up time. Over-arousal takes up some of our ability to process things as we usually might and to remain calm and focussed. It pushes aside our capacity to continue to function as we might otherwise and to engage in the core behaviours of eating, drinking, sleeping, and thinking.

Difficulties with arousal levels are very common in children with ARFID. We have previously noted in the discussion on *correlates* (Chapter 2: Who can develop ARFID?) that the neurodevelopmental conditions autism and ADHD often co-occur. Over-arousal or over-stimulation is certainly a shared characteristic. Many autistic children have heightened sensitivity to a range of stimuli. They can also become quite fixated on patterns of movement or particular sounds. Some become extremely distressed by specific textures or noises, others may smell or feel everything. This does not always affect their eating to an extreme degree but in some children, like Samir, it does.

Samir is a nine-year-old boy with significant autism. He does not communicate with speech, but will often make a range of sounds that his parents describe as expressing his mood.

Samir loves music and has two favourite tunes which he never tires of hearing. He likes to move his upper body and arms when the music plays. Samir's parents describe him as a contented child as long as there are no surprises.

Samir attends a school that caters for the needs of children with autism. He seems generally settled and happy there and as long as his routine is not changed he manages reasonably well. On the days something unpredictable happens, Samir can become very distressed and has a tendency to hit out. This can be triggered by a loud noise outside, another child becoming upset and shouting, or by someone bumping into him. He also finds it very difficult to be in the playground when other children are running about. He prefers to stand behind the big tree where he can't see them and stroke its bark. Although the staff are very good at helping him to manage the day at school, his parents will often receive a call from the school to say he has hit someone. Samir's school has a sensory room, which is a quiet space with coloured lights and toys that Samir likes to spin and watch. This will sometimes help him to become a bit calmer, but if he has become very distressed, this might not work as well.

One area that is a significant difficulty is getting Samir to eat anything at all at school. At home, his parents manage to get him to eat his preferred pureed food by sticking to exactly the same routine and playing a song that they call the eating song. Although they have heard it hundreds of times, it seems to help Samir know it is time to eat and he allows his mother to support him eating while he watches his tablet. Samir's parents described being very concerned that at nine years of age he is unable to eat anything without support, and does not eat anything at all during the school day. His mother was embarrassed to report that he was still on the same toddler foods he had been eating for years. They had worked hard to ensure he continued to gain weight and grow by increasing the amounts of these foods and by giving him chocolate buttons which he liked to suck. Samir's father said that they were now spending large amounts of money and having to bulk buy his preferred foods. His mother said she knew he wasn't getting the nutrition that he needed but did not know what else she could do.

Samir was unable to manage the combined demands of noise, smell, and movement at school at the same time as putting anything in his mouth. Altogether this represented an overload of stimulation, sending his arousal levels up to a level that he could not cope with. The over-arousal from the busy lunchtime setting meant that Samir simply did not have enough capacity to process all the sensory input and was unable to engage in eating. Consequently, his intake was inadequate to meet his nutritional needs. This is seen, perhaps to a lesser extent, in many children on the autism spectrum. If the effect on eating results in the levels of impairment we discussed in the chapter on *characteristics* (Chapter 1: What is ARFID?) then it requires attention and should not simply be considered 'part of the autism'.

In ADHD, arousal levels are typically high, in particular when there is a strong component of hyperactivity or impulsivity. Some children with ADHD seem too busy to eat. They can be extremely active and find it very difficult to sit down at the table. Things other than food and mealtimes are much more compelling; attention is constantly diverted to multiple things simultaneously, making it hard for them to focus on or pay attention to any one thing, in this case eating. The low interest in food and eating seen in children with ARFID in the context of ADHD may be related to this over-arousal. As with autism however, not all children with ADHD have significant eating difficulties.

Habitual undereating

It might seem rather counter-intuitive that undereating can be associated with a reduced desire to eat. Occasional undereating usually has the opposite effect. If most of us have been delayed having a meal or had to manage on only a small amount of food for one reason or another, we are certainly ready to eat as soon as the next opportunity arises! This is the body sending appropriate signals to let us know that re-fuelling is required. However, things are rather different in the case of habitual undereating, which is often related to lowered appetite. There are a number of possible reasons why this might be the case. Firstly, when someone does not eat enough, they generally tend to become tired and irritable. Mood may be affected and hunger can be blunted. Another common effect of undereating is the tendency to become constipated. Constipation can be uncomfortable with abdominal bloating and a feeling of fullness which can also put people off eating. In the case of habitual undereating, the body seems to slow down and to manage on what it receives, sending only weak signals to say feed me. People sometimes say things like 'She has been eating like a bird and her stomach has shrunk'. Of course stomachs do not really shrink, but if they are constantly given a small amount of food, they demand less. In this situation someone might feel full, or at least satisfied enough to make them stop eating, after only a very small amount. This is quite common in children with ARFID who have very restricted intake. They will make clear they have had enough after only a few mouthfuls and will push food away. They are rarely hungry and do not usually ask for food. Thankfully, just as the stomach adapts to having too little, it can be retrained to accept greater quantities. We will revisit this in the chapters on *care* (Chapter 5: What can I do? and Chapter 6: What is the best treatment for ARFID?).

Oral-motor or swallowing difficulties

For the sake of completeness in terms of our consideration of why someone might have low interest in food we also need to consider the possibility that eating is hard work or uncomfortable in some way. If these are the only reasons there are eating difficulties and they can be corrected so that any avoidance or restriction disappears, then we are not talking about ARFID. For example if someone has a really persistent, painful throat infection so that all they can eat is ice cream or yoghurt, we would anticipate that once effectively treated, eating would pick up. Similarly a child with diagnosed swallow dysfunction (or dysphagia) might experience discomfort swallowing certain textures which is likely to put them off. Dysphagia is often present in children with a range of developmental and genetic conditions; in most instances medically recommended avoidance of certain textures can be managed without compromising the child's intake or interest in food or eating. However, there are some children with ARFID who do struggle more with certain textures, or with biting and chewing, which can put them off eating more generally. These difficulties can be related to structural issues or to lack of practice, but the key is that in the child with ARFID the effect will have been to put them off eating more generally. We have seen plenty of children in clinic, who do struggle with chewy foods but are regularly sitting in front of foods that are simply too difficult, too tiring or require too much effort for them to manage. It seems little wonder that such children may end up with low interest in food or eating. It is also potentially dangerous, as they may not have sufficiently well-developed oral-motor skills to manage large lumps that may break off which can lead to gagging and choking. Unsurprisingly, this reinforces the reluctance to eat.

Related to a medical condition or illness

Everyone knows that being unwell is often associated with lowered interest in eating. Many of us go off our food if we are battling an infection, or are under the weather. Sometimes we restrict our eating to a few, usually bland, foods we feel comfortable with. Some medical conditions are associated with the need to put specific recommendations around eating in place or to restrict certain foods in the diet, for example, insulin-dependent diabetes or coeliac disease. Avoidance and restriction in these cases are medically prescribed and directly related to a medical condition; this is not ARFID. In most instances, the person's eating pattern will accommodate the exclusions and restrictions without undue negative impact.

In our discussion on *correlates* (Chapter 2: Who can develop ARFID?), we have seen that ARFID can occur alongside a range of medical conditions. However, we also know from the sections on *characteristics* (Chapter 1: What is ARFID?) that the eating difficulty should be over and above that usually explained by the illness or condition, if a diagnosis of ARFID is to be considered. There are certainly children with ARFID who have either complex medical histories, or ongoing conditions, where this is certainly the case. The relationship between the two may be influenced by persisting low interest in eating, originally stemming from the illness, but is more likely to stem from negative associations with food or eating, as with Jessica.

Jessica had been on holiday with her family when she picked up a nasty gastrointestinal infection. Up until that point, the family had been enjoying their holiday abroad in the sunshine. Jessica had been swimming every day, making friends with other children on holiday and enjoying trying different types of food. Unfortunately she developed severe vomiting and diarrhoea and became floppy and dehydrated. Her parents tried to care for her in their holiday villa but as she failed to improve they sought local medical advice. Jessica was taken to the local hospital and admitted. She was very clingy and frightened as she couldn't understand what anyone was saying. Jessica had always been terrified of needles but she was so poorly that she had to have a drip. She was sure that the food she had been eating had made her so ill.

Long after the infection cleared up and she had no other symptoms she continued to show low interest in food and eating. Her parents described her as previously having been a good eater and could not understand why she was not returning to her old self. Jessica understood that the food she might eat at home or at school would be no more likely to make her ill than it ever had, and said she was not frightened of eating. She was able to explain that the main problem was that every time she sat down to eat or put something in her mouth, all sorts of memories came flooding back of the hospital, the beeping drip, and how horrible it had all been. Food and mealtimes were no longer something to be enjoyed.

Related to being on certain medications

The final reason someone may have low interest in eating that we will consider here, is because they are taking certain medications. A number of pills and medicines have the effect of reducing (or in some cases increasing) appetite, as a side effect, alongside acting in the manner intended. Drugs known to reduce appetite as a side effect include some of those used in the treatment of a wide range of conditions, including asthma, cancer, ulcerative colitis, and ADHD. There are many examples. Usually individuals prescribed medications known to suppress appetite will be monitored for weight loss, and steps taken to minimise the impact of this effect. Some children with ARFID and co-occurring medical conditions are on medications known to impair appetite; however in almost all, there will be other factors at play that contribute to the avoidance or restriction. The effect of the medication is better considered as an additional hurdle to overcome rather than a cause of the ARFID.

Avoidance based on sensory aspects of food or eating

By comparison with the discussion above of avoidance or restriction of food or eating being related to low interest, avoidance related to sensory experience seems rather more straightforward! We have already established in reviewing the *characteristics* of ARFID (Chapter 1: What is ARFID?) that sensory sensitivities and preferences are well documented as playing a role in avoidance or restriction in many. Indeed, they are given as an example in the diagnostic criteria. We have also established that one particular *correlate* (Chapter 2: Who can develop ARFID?), autism, often shares unusual sensory reactivity or highly specific sensory interests with features associated with ARFID. So how exactly does sensory sensitivity *cause* problems with eating behaviour?

We interact with our environment using our five senses: sight, smell, hearing, taste, and touch. Some of us have more acute senses in one or more of these avenues of perception than others. One person might have 'a good nose' and another might be able to hear pitches and tones that the person next to them can't. Our responses to the input we receive and process using our senses are on a continuum from very pleasant to very unpleasant. We might really like a painting, find a piece of music very soothing, or enjoy the soft feeling of a new jumper when our sensory responses are on the pleasant side of the spectrum. On the unpleasant side, we can find smells off-putting, the sight of a dead mouse revolting, or turn off the radio because a song is too jangly. One emotion that is often associated with this unpleasant side is disgust. Disgust is a fascinating emotion, thought to originate from the need for humans to be put off things that might be dangerous. It is a strong emotion which often leads us to pull a highly specific 'disgust face' (try it – it is different from your other facial expressions!). Disgust goes hand in hand with pulling back and avoiding things. From an evolutionary perspective, you can see it might come in handy.

In ARFID, and in particular in relation to avoidance and restriction based on sensory aspects of food or eating, disgust often plays a significant role. Children will complain loudly that anything other than their preferred foods looks/feels/smells disgusting, revolting, and gross. If they get as far as tasting, it may be spat out, lead to gagging (or even vomiting), tears or rage, and statements about never, ever eating that again! Disgust is at play and, as we have seen, most of us respond to this by avoidance. Your child is behaving like a human being and refusing. The disgust response is causing a rise in alertness to danger. This does not necessarily have to go along with consciously thinking something will be dangerous to eat; this process occurs naturally. The problem here is that acute sensitivity to differences in the taste, sight, smell, texture, temperature or sound of food triggers the disgust response very easily so that we end up with avoidance and refusal. It can also be the case that even a couple of early experiences which have led to a disgust response can make a child very wary of trying anything that does not look or smell right, or is in a different packet. They might not even get as far as tasting or touching and you are left with the 'stuck' diets that many parents of children with ARFID (including Hallie's, whom we met in Chapter 1) are very familiar with.

Avoidance related to concern about possible negative consequences of eating

Just as the above section was largely about one emotion, disgust, in relation to sensory experience, this section is largely about another emotion, fear, in relation to previous experience. As with disgust, fear is an essential emotion and from an evolutionary perspective is vital for survival. If you didn't feel fear in the presence of a large, snarling, hungry carnivore running towards you, you might not last long. When humans experience fear, all sort of things happen in the body; it becomes more alert and ready to act. Sometimes you can 'read' fear in someone else, not only by their facial expression (very different to the 'disgust face'), but also by their breathing, their face changing colour, their pupils getting bigger, or by shaking. The terrified person is likely to feel their heart thumping and may become sweaty. All these things are in response to hormones that are released when we experience fear that get the body ready for what is often known as the fight or flight response: I am either going to stand my ground and fight the charging beast with everything I have got or I am going to run away to safety as quickly as I can. In relation to our discussion here, this roughly translates to: I am going to stand my ground and refuse to try anything different despite your repeated attempts or I am going to make sure I avoid any possible chance of having something that isn't what I feel safe with.

So let's explore common fear-driven causes of avoidance and restriction in children a little more. Why does this happen? There can be a number of reasons, some related to things that have happened to the child, that is, within their own direct experience, and some related to things they may have learned or picked up from others, that is, through indirect experience. If any of us has had a nasty or unpleasant experience which has been associated with being frightened, we will generally want to avoid that in the future. Although the fear response makes sense for humans, it isn't generally experienced as a pleasant thing. A number of the children we have met already have had difficult early medical histories. Medical intervention in the early years can have different effects on children, we think in part due to their temperament. A temperamentally anxious child may experience more fear related to procedures than a more confident, adventurous one. Very early adverse experiences related to food or eating may in some children continue to contribute to fear related to food or eating, even after many years. Some children with significant allergies may refuse a much wider range of foods than they need to exclude from their diet for medical reasons, due to concern about what might happen to them. Of course there are also other reasons in children who do not have complex medical histories, such as a choking episode, a really bad bout of gastroenteritis, a sensation of not being able to breathe, a fear of being poisoned, all of which may elicit a fear response at the time which then remains in place and generalises much more widely. Emmie, whom we met in Chapter 1, is an example of this.

Indirect experience can also contribute to fear-based avoidance and restriction. Kelsey and Lewis's examples illustrate this.

Kelsey was an only child who lived with her single mother. Her parents had separated when she was a baby and her father now had a new family. Kelsey was very attached to her mother, and the two of them spent a lot of time together. Kelsey's mother had features of obsessive compulsive disorder (OCD). She had never been formally diagnosed, but she was very concerned about germs and spent a significant part of each day cleaning the flat while Kelsey was at school. Kelsey's mother repeatedly reminded her to wash her hands, and Kelsey would help with the cleaning at weekends. She had become increasingly worried about germs on her food.

Kelsey first attended the clinic at the age of seven years. She appeared a shy, anxious child, and was very clingy towards her mother. It became clear that there was a strong element of dependence on each other. Kelsey slept with her mother at night, which seemed to be something they both felt safer with. When her mother brought her to clinic, Kelsey was only eating food from sealed packets or containers. She refused anything from an open packet, expressing concern that germs might have got in. Kelsey had not had any negative experiences herself from food that had gone off or had been contaminated in any way. She had learned to fear germs in particular from her mother, with a temperament that made her particularly vulnerable to worrying about things.

Lewis was a ten-year-old boy whose father had severe allergies. His father was a larger than life, cheerful character who had a good friendship network. Lewis was the youngest child of his parents, living with them and his two older sisters. The family was a close one, with all members getting on well. When on an outing with his father, Lewis had witnessed his father having an allergic reaction to something he had eaten at a café where they had lunch. His father needed to use an epipen, which he carried with him in case of such an event. Lewis had been terrified and thought his father was dying. He was scared not only that his father might die, but also did not know what he would do as he was far from home. His father recovered quite quickly, but since this event, Lewis started to become very worried about him and about what his father might eat when Lewis was at school. Over time his anxiety became so great that his own eating became affected. When he came to clinic, Lewis was very tearful and felt he had to be extremely cautious not only about his own eating, but also about what everyone else was eating. Lewis had not had any bad experiences related to food and eating himself, but witnessing his father's adverse reaction and believing he was going to die, had eventually led to Lewis restricting his own intake.

In this chapter we have considered a very wide range of factors that may contribute to the development of ARFID. We have seen that the most appropriate answer to the question 'Why does someone develop ARFID?' is likely to be 'It depends!' We have explored things that can influence our interest in food and eating and whether the experience of eating is pleasant or off-putting. We have considered things that might shape our thoughts and beliefs as we sit down to a meal or think about eating. We have thought about disgust and fear and their role in leading to avoidance and restriction. It is likely that some, but not all, of these things might strike a chord with you as you consider your own child's eating. We have also thought about the complex nature of determining causality, 'What *causes* ARFID?', and concluded that at present it seems sensible to think that it can have multiple contributing factors, which tend to vary between individuals. As you think about the *cause* of ARFID in relation to your own child's situation, it is perhaps best to approach this as an exercise aimed at trying to understand why things are the way they are. It is rarely helpful to get into a way of thinking along the lines of fault, blame or regret. We will return to this in the first of our *care* chapters (Chapter 5: What can I do?), as well as consider how we can intervene to change things in our second care chapter (Chapter 6: What is the best treatment for ARFID?). For now we will move on to considering what happens to someone who develops ARFID; what are the *consequences*?

Chapter 4

What are the consequences of having ARFID?

This chapter will cover the possible *consequences* or impact of having ARFID, on the individual concerned as well as on others, including family members. We will focus particularly on the impact of ARFID in children and young people. This is not intended to be a chapter that causes alarm, as it is very unlikely that all possible areas of impact are present in any one child and family. You may recognise some as being present, but only to a minor degree, whereas others may be major sources of concern for you. As parents and carers, your role is to make informed decisions in your child's best interests. This includes making decisions about your own strategies and priorities in trying to help your child as well as decisions made together with health care staff about treatment. This chapter will therefore set out the full range of areas of possible impact, so that you can approach your decision making with knowledge about the possible risks of avoidance and restriction related to your child's eating. We will move on to what can be done to address these areas of impact in the two chapters discussing *care* (Chapter 5: What can I do? and Chapter 6: What is the best treatment for ARFID?).

The most obvious place to start is by discussing the four areas that form part of the definition of ARFID and already referred to in the section on *characteristics* (Chapter 1: What is ARFID?). You will recall that we saw that the avoidance or restriction of food intake may lead to one or more of four things: weight or growth problems; nutritional deficiency; dependence on tube feeding or nutritional supplements; interference with everyday functioning. Let's consider the possible consequences of each in turn, in a bit more detail.

Weight or growth problems

We all need to eat, to provide our body with the energy it needs to function properly. We use up most of our energy resting, sleeping, keeping warm, and just being alive. Our brain uses energy thinking and every organ of our body needs energy to keep it working. We need some energy to help us digest food, and we need energy to allow us to move about and engage in activities. The term usually used for the units of energy released from food is 'calories'. Insufficient energy intake is the same as saying insufficient calorie intake. If we don't eat enough calories to keep us going, we tend to feel weak, tired, and irritable. We may struggle to concentrate and feel light-headed. We may struggle to sleep. If there is a sustained failure to eat the amount of calories our body needs, we might lose weight as we have caused an energy deficit. The problem, as many dieters will know, is that our bodies tend to adjust to not being given quite enough, and start to use less energy to keep things going. This is the commonly experienced plateau effect in deliberate efforts to lose weight, as seen in dieting. There might be an initial drop in weight, but it gets harder to lose more as the body compensates, and many people give up.

The amount of energy we need can vary depending on what we are doing; if we are more active, we need more calories. Mostly these adjustments happen quite naturally as long as our hunger signals are working properly. For example, if you have been for an energetic swim you may feel hungry afterwards; your body needs a top-up after all the energy it has used in the pool. Polar explorers provide an extreme example of differences in energy needs depending on what they are doing. While they are in the initial stages of planning their trip, sitting at the computer making lists, maps, and calculations, there is no real need to change their usual diet and calorie intake. As they begin to prepare and to improve their stamina and fitness, their energy needs will increase. When they are on the expedition, in freezing weather and engaging in strenuous physical activity, their energy needs can shoot up to more than three times what they would otherwise need. That is a lot of calories to eat! Imagine eating the equivalent of three breakfasts, three lunches and three dinners plus three times the snacks you would normally have, and having to do that every day. Many polar explorers return having lost a lot of weight as their daily intake has been less than their body has been using up each day.

The human body can vary a great detail in its energy needs, both between individuals and, as we have seen, in relation to what any one person is doing. Some people naturally use up more energy from their food than others. They may be described as having a higher metabolism. Such people might find it much harder to put on weight than others, and conversely may lose it more easily, for example, due to a bout of illness. It is not yet fully understood why there are such differences, but we probably all know people who struggle to put weight on, or those who seem to put it on very easily, even if they are eating the same amount as someone who does not.

The situation with children is slightly different; as they grow they need to increase their energy intake to see them through all the demands of their development. Healthy children should be increasing their weight at a rate in line with the tracks on a growth chart. Most parents will be familiar with these. When children are young, weight measurements tend to be plotted as a dot on the chart. The child may be checked to see that their weight is increasing as expected over time. If children are not taking in enough calories and this persists over a period of time, this may impact not only weight but their growth as well. In children with ARFID who have insufficient energy intake, weight can remain static or it might actually drop. It is important to recognise that the absence of weight increase in a child who is not overweight is already equivalent to an adult dropping weight. If they have a loss of weight in real terms, the urgency to address this is greater than in an adult. In extreme cases this can lead to what is sometimes referred to as 'wasting'. There are formal definitions for this term, but essentially it means that the child's weight is much lower than it should be for their height and they generally look unhealthily thin. When the normal pattern of weight gain is negatively affected, the rate at which the child is growing also tends to slow down and they may stay the same height for much longer than is usual. In extreme cases this can lead to what is known as 'stunting'. Again, there are technical definitions for this term, but essentially it means that the child will be smaller than the majority of their peers and fail to grow in the way that would normally be expected. Together, this negative impact on weight and growth is sometimes called 'faltering growth'.

It is important to be clear that not all children with ARFID fail to eat enough in terms of calories. Many will meet or even exceed their calorie requirements, so this may not be an issue you are concerned about in relation to your own child. If it is something relevant to your own situation, you may be aware that energy deficits in children can not only affect weight and height, but also mean that there is less energy available to keep the body going and to have left over to sustain development. Children with inadequate calorie intake may find it hard to concentrate as their brain is unable to access the energy it needs. This can impact on learning. Their behaviour can also be adversely affected, and they may become tetchy or tearful. They may be tired all the time and unable to take part in the normal range of age-appropriate activities. In short, inadequate energy intake over a prolonged period is not good for children and when this occurs, it needs to be addressed.

Nutritional inadequacies or deficiencies

Avoidance and restriction of food intake can result in too little being eaten overall, as above, or it can result in too few of some foods being eaten, leading to an unbalanced diet. In the discussion on *characteristics* (Chapter 1: What is ARFID?), the terms micronutrients and macronutrients were used in relation to a healthy diet. Micronutrients are the vitamins and minerals present in many foods, usually in only small amounts, but nonetheless an essential part of a balanced diet that meets the body's needs. Macronutrients are the major food groups, such as carbohydrates, fats, proteins, which we need in larger amounts and are equally important to include in the diet. Together the micro- and macronutrient profile of any one person's diet will play a part in their general health and well-being, and in children, also their development. Good nutrition makes us feel better and allows us to function better.

The body's needs for these nutrients change with age and stage of development, with most requirements rising steadily throughout childhood and through adolescence. Some children with ARFID may struggle to increase their intake of certain foods in line with their needs, while others may avoid entire food groups. Most countries publish national guidelines for recommended intake of different nutrients, with most stating that under normal circumstances requirements should ideally be met through the diet. Exceptions to this are some of the recommendations for very young children; in the UK for example, the current government recommendation is that all children under the age of five years should have their food and fluid intake supplemented by vitamin A, C, and D drops. It can be difficult for us all as parents to get the balance right in our attempts to make sure our children are getting what they need. It is not the intention that people should spend hours doing complex calculations or weighing or measuring their children's food. General guidance about macronutrients in the form of a balanced diet, if followed, will generally suffice. Recommendations and dietary guidelines are put in place to limit the likelihood of people developing nutritional deficiencies, which may be harmful to health and development.

This is not intended to be a nutrition handbook and so an exhaustive list of all the possible consequences of inadequate nutritional intake is not included here. In children with ARFID some of the more commonly encountered consequences are iron deficiencies leading to anaemia, calcium and vitamin D deficiencies leading to poor bone health and rickets, vitamin A deficiency leading to eye and skin problems, and in some cases vitamin C deficiency leading to scurvy. Deficiencies at this level represent serious problems that can impair children's health and certainly require attention.

As with insufficient energy intake, inadequate nutritional intake can not only have a direct impact, here in terms of deficiencies expressed as physical conditions, it can also have a wider impact on development and everyday functioning. Good nutrition is important for brain development and throughout childhood and adolescence, your child's brain is constantly developing. Although the human brain is actually remarkably resistant and able to survive periods of quite poor nutrition, specific deficiencies can cause difficulties and hamper learning and functioning. Most parents are keen that their children have the nutrition they need to develop to their full potential and so this is often a concern for parents of children with ARFID.

Dependence on tube feeds or nutritional supplements

We have seen that persistent poor eaters who are failing to meet energy and/or nutritional needs may be started on tube feeds. As mentioned in the discussion about *characteristics* (Chapter 1: What is ARFID?), this may be via a nasogastric tube, a gastrostomy tube (a PEG), or via a tube that goes into the small intestine (the jejunum; a PEG-J), depending on the individual circumstances. The decision to proceed with tube feeding is usually made following discussion with the child's caregivers on the basis that it is considered medically necessary at the time to sustain the child's nutritional and energy needs. Used in this way, tube feeding can without doubt be in the child's best interests, and in some cases is life-saving. It may be necessary to move from one form of tube feeding to another if the initial route is not tolerated, or if the child continues to make little progress with eating and drinking. Decisions to change the type of tube feeding are also usually made by health care professionals together with the parents, taking the child's medical needs and best interests into account.

Why do children become dependent on tube feeds? Why do they continue to rely on being fed by this route when it is no longer medically necessary? Leaving aside those children who are physically unable to eat adequately (in other words those who can't eat enough, rather than those who won't eat enough), let us try to address this question. There are a number of possible reasons. At the time a tube goes in, families are usually experiencing a high degree of stress trying to feed a child who is refusing to eat and clearly struggling physically. This can be hugely worrying and upsetting as well as at times being very frustrating. Many parents describe having to think long and hard about agreeing to tube feeding, as this is something they might prefer to avoid. Often they feel that they have tried everything and nothing is working and so they agree on the basis that they can see no other option. Other parents may feel relieved at the prospect of a tube as they feel overwhelmed with worry about their child's health and well-being and want to take positive action. Initially, if it has been agreed to tube feed, most children will start on a nasogastric tube. Sometimes this can be experienced as uncomfortable, but the majority of children will quickly get used to the tube and are able to receive much better nutrition than has been previously possible. As a consequence, everyone can relax a little. It may be inconvenient, but many parents describe an overwhelming feeling of relief that their child is being fed adequately. Under usual circumstances, the child will begin to feel better, appetite picks up and they become more amenable to taking food by mouth. This is the most common situation in children who need tube feeding in the context of an episode of illness.

Sometimes dependency on tube feeds is a relatively straightforward matter of the child not really having an opportunity to become hungry enough to want to eat. If all their nutritional needs are met via the feed going down the tube, the body's natural tendency to self-regulate will mean that no signals are given to make the child want to eat. Under normal circumstances, this can be managed by spacing out the tube feeds or by dropping one and trying to create times of the day when the child is more likely to feel hungry. Alternatively, the overall amount of tube feed may be reduced so that self-regulation kicks in and the child compensates by eating more.

In children with ARFID the situation is often different. These children will have been refusing food or struggling to eat, not because they are feeling very unwell, but because they are not interested, can't stand the texture, are frightened of the food, or another of the reasons we are now familiar with. They may indeed feel physically better or put on weight through tube feeding, but that does not address the underlying difficulties. Continuing to offer such children foods as before is likely to continue to be met with refusal, and any attempts to wean them off the tube seem to fail. When nasogastric feeding has been in place for three months or so, the usual guidance is that consideration should be given to stop this form of feeding, or if this is not possible, to consider whether a move to gastrostomy feeding is needed. The placement of a gastrostomy tube requires surgical intervention, which means that parents or carers will need to provide consent on their child's behalf when they are too young to do so. Again, the majority of parents do their best to proceed in the best interests of their child and sometimes there can seem no other alternative in the face of ongoing avoidance and refusal, even though the child may be in a better state physically.

Once the gastrostomy tube is in place, there tends to be greater flexibility around feeding patterns. Some children are fed using a pump overnight. The feed dispenser fits onto the tube going into their stomach. The pump can be turned on to a steady rate so the child gets fed a specified amount during the night. The pump will beep when it is finished and needs switching off, or if something goes wrong. Threading the pipe up through a pyjama leg helps to avoid tangling and most children are not disturbed during the feed. Other children may be fed during the day, more or less following a mealtime pattern, again using a pump or using a special syringe. Some children are fed both during the day and overnight. Most families slot into a routine of tube feeding and the child's nutrition is taken care of.

The problem here is that routines are usually habit forming. Tube feeding has in many instances been such a positive move in terms of the child's health and in terms of relieving stress that it is not hard to see why it might become established. Ideally, when a tube is placed via whatever route, it should go along with a plan to help the child move away from needing tube feeding. In children with ARFID, this often requires something other than continuing to present the child with previously rejected foods or manipulating the feeding pattern to try to create windows of hunger. If their eating behaviour is driven by low interest, disgust or fear, this alone can't be expected to help a great deal. We will look at what can be done in the discussion on *care* (Chapter 6: What is the best treatment for ARFID?).

For the sake of completeness, it may be worth considering why children may become dependent on tube feeding via the jejunum, or feeding via a PEG-J. This would be more unusual than gastrostomy feeding and is generally used for people with significant gastrointestinal conditions who are unable to tolerate food in the stomach. We know that a few children with ARFID, such as John, end up being fed by PEG-J and becoming quite stuck on this form of feeding.

> John is 13 years old, the only child of his parents, who themselves are both only children. John's mother was 39 years old when she had John, and his parents are now aged 52 and 56 respectively. They are a churchgoing family and most of their social contact is via their local church community. John is now nearing the end of his second year at senior school, but his attendance over the past year has been very poor due to him being unwell. He does not particularly enjoy going to school as he finds it hard to fit in with most of the other students. He experienced some teasing in his first year, which upset him greatly. John described liking a few of the teachers and when his school attendance had been better, he preferred to spend his break time joining one of the lunchtime clubs run by the staff in the Science Department. When they attend the clinic, John and his parents appear very close. They are all extremely concerned about what has happened to John.
>
> They describe John having been badly winded playing football at school in the summer of his first year. He and a much larger boy had collided and John had felt he could not breathe. He had been terrified that he might die. When he got his breath back he became very tearful, made worse by the sports teacher telling him to 'man up' and a number of the other children laughing at him. On return home John told his mother that he had had an accident at school and had thought he might die. His mother called the school, but they did not appear to have any record of anything untoward. The school later called back to confirm that John had indeed had

a minor bump on the football pitch but that it was nothing out of the ordinary and he was completely unharmed.

John slept badly that night, lying awake concentrating on his breathing. He felt unable to go to school the next day, which was a Friday, and stayed at home with his mother. He continued to focus on his breathing over the weekend. On his return to school on the Monday, on entering the dining room, he became extremely anxious that he might not be able breathe properly at the same time as eating his lunch. He took his tray to the table but was unable to eat anything more than a few nibbles. Over time the situation worsened, with John only able to eat soft foods that he could swallow quickly when at home, and unable to eat at all at school. John's parents described him starting to lose weight, which became even worse when the whole family went down with a vomiting bug his father had picked up at work. After this John seemed unable to keep anything down at all, long after the bug had cleared up. John was terrified that he had suffered some lasting damage and would die. Understandably his parents were extremely concerned; he was constantly being sick, complaining of feeling unwell and being unable to breathe properly, and looked dreadful.

The dietitian suggested some fortified drinks to build him up, but John could not contemplate taking these as he was convinced they would make him even sicker. He did try some and was promptly sick which he said proved his point. Eventually, the situation got so bad that he was admitted to hospital and a nasogastric tube was passed. By this time he was due to go back to school to start his second year but was unable to do so. Over the following two terms things went from bad to worse. John had a number of investigations and nothing untoward was ever identified. This did not seem to reassure him and the sickness continued whenever he tried to eat anything other than yoghurts or ice cream. Eventually he had surgery to have a gastrostomy tube placed. He continued to refuse almost all foods and complained that the feed was harming him and making him sick. The medical team and John's parents came to the conclusion that his stomach needed a rest and so a period of feeding directly into his small intestine was the only option to try to get some nutrition into him and to help restore some weight. John remained terrified but agreed there was nothing else to be done.

When he came to the clinic, John's vomiting had stopped and his weight was better than it had been. He had missed a significant amount of school and was dependent on the PEG-J for his nutrition. He was tolerating small amounts of a limited range of soft foods and was able to suck pieces of chocolate. He was avoiding most foods on the grounds that he would not be able to manage them. His parents were exhausted and distraught.

John's situation is quite extreme but perhaps understandable in the context of his fears and experience. The impact on the whole family was significant. Dependence on tube feeds can be difficult to manage and when present to this degree, takes a lot of time and effort on everybody's part. Thankfully however, it is possible to manage; John was eventually able to return to normal eating (described in Chapter 6: What is the best treatment for ARFID?).

As well as dependence on tube feeds, it is also possible that children with ARFID develop a dependence on nutritional supplements. This term is used here to include specially formulated drinks that contain both calories and a wide range of nutrients. These are often the same feeds that are administered via a tube. There are a range of such supplement feeds available and they may be prescribed for children who for one reason or another are not taking in enough energy and whose overall intake is inadequate. There are two other related types of product, also usually prescribed by the doctor or a dietitian; one that can be used to boost calorie intake alone and the other to improve the nutritional profile of existing intake, sometimes in a powder form. The calorie boosters may be used in children whose overall intake is meeting their nutritional requirements but who just do not eat enough to meet their energy needs. These supplements primarily consist of fats and sugars which are high in calories. The powders may be used for children who are meeting their energy requirements but the diet is very limited and so their overall nutrition is very poor.

They do not need extra calories, but do need help to improve their intake. The powder is generally mixed with food or drinks and added in this way. Just as with tube feeds, the use of such prescribed products can be extremely helpful. The extra calories can help with weight gain, and the vitamins, minerals and other trace elements they contain can help address any nutritional inadequacies. They will generally be prescribed when this is medically necessary. However, also just as with the tube feeds, many children remain 'stuck' on these supplements. The fortified drinks may be preferred by the child and experienced as easier to take than food. Supplements that take care of all the child's nutritional needs may seem much easier to take than eating fruit, vegetables, and a range of other foods that would otherwise be needed.

There is another important reason why children might become stuck on supplements. Many are quite energy dense, that is, they contain a lot of calories (which is after all the point). This means that they can take a while to digest and tend to sit in the stomach. This can have the effect of dampening hunger. In some cases putting children on supplements can even reduce their food intake. A number of similar products can be purchased without a prescription. These are intended to be given in addition to the child's usual intake and may for example be helpful if a child has been unwell and needs a bit of help. However we know that a number of parents report that they result in their child not being hungry at mealtimes and ending up eating less.

Supplements can therefore be helpful in the short term but it is not difficult to see why many children with ARFID may come to depend on them. It is also not difficult to see why many parents might be relieved their child takes them, as this way their nutrition is assured. Moving away from using them once weight and nutrition have been improved can be difficult. Again the underlying drivers of their food avoidance and refusal are not addressed through their use.

Interference with everyday functioning

The fourth major area of impact of ARFID includes a wide range of possible consequences in terms of everyday functioning. These can be separated into consequences for the child and consequences for the family. We asked parents and carers attending our clinic if they could tell us what the main areas of impact of ARFID were in their situation. Leaving aside the consequences for the child's health and growth which we have discussed above, they came up with the following list of things they felt were negatively affected:

- the child's social life
- the child's mood
- the child's energy levels and stamina
- the child's learning

as well as:

- family mealtimes
- their own anxiety levels as parents
- their other children's anxiety levels
- their own or their partner's mood
- their other children's behaviour
- their relationship as parents
- their confidence in their own parenting abilities
- family finances
- their ability to travel/go away on holiday
- their social life

Do you recognise any of these? Perhaps you recognise all of them. They are certainly things that we see very often in families with a child with ARFID. Children may be unable to participate in normal age-appropriate activities or opportunities that are open to their peers. They may miss out on things like sitting with class mates at lunchtime or going to a birthday party. They may miss out on school trips, sleepovers, or staying with relatives – all really important aspects of children developing independence. They may be too tired, afraid, overwhelmed or stressed to be able to join in. This can impact negatively on their social and emotional development as they may have fewer opportunities to negotiate normal developmental tasks and demands. Over time, they may become more socially isolated or subjected to teasing. They may become unhappy. They may struggle to manage their behaviour, with loud displays of distress, frustration or anger when out, because the situation is too challenging for them. They may fall out with their siblings. They may not be able to eat anywhere other than at home. Some children with ARFID may develop a self-identity as a person who just does not eat a wide range of foods, seeming to retreat into the safety of being very clear and consistent in their refusal and having limited or no expectation that anything will change, or indeed needs to change. Of course, not all these things will be present in all children with ARFID.

In terms of the consequences of ARFID on family life, as you can see from the list above, they can be significant and far reaching. Families often make adjustments to try to accommodate their child's difficulty, but this can become more difficult as time goes by. Some parents describe driving round a number of shops and supermarkets trying to buy the one particular flavour of the one particular brand of one particular type of food that their child is relying on. The toll on parents and other members on the family can be profound. ARFID can cause stress as well as distress, and can affect every family member in one way or another. It can lead parents to behave in ways they wouldn't usually, sometimes crying or shouting through worry and frustration or overcompensating to protect their child from becoming upset. A common issue described by parents is the effect on the behaviour of other children in the family. They may complain that it is unfair that their brother or sister always gets certain foods they would like, such as chips; start to refuse foods they have previously eaten; or act the fool or misbehave at the table to get your attention because you seem to be giving it all to their sibling. You may feel undermined, defeated, and at the end of your tether, with mealtimes a complete nightmare and no prospect of being able to eat anywhere else. Your mental health may be negatively affected; you argue with your partner, feel useless as a parent and have a permanent sense of helplessness and hopelessness. You may withdraw from your own friends, who really do not seem to understand, or limit conversation with your own relatives who do not seem to want to help.

Clearly there are many different ways ARFID can have an impact on everyday functioning; for your child, for you, and for others in your family. It is absolutely not the intention that reading about all these possible negative consequences should increase your anxiety or make you feel even gloomier than when you picked up this book. It is extremely important to recognise that all these areas of impact can be addressed. This chapter can therefore serve as a means of checking in with yourself what the impact of your child's eating currently is on each person in your own family. Really think about it, and write it down. Talk about it with your partner, and if appropriate, with your other children to check what their experience is. That way you can formulate a plan of action. In our next chapter on *care* (Chapter 5: What can I do?) we will begin to think about what that might look like.

Chapter 5

What can I do?

This is an important chapter. As a parent you are likely to have picked up this book because you want to find out more about ARFID, but just as much – and if not more – because you actively want to *do* something. Either to do something to help your child, who may be clearly experiencing difficulties with their eating, or to do something to prevent what you suspect are emerging difficulties or signs of ARFID, from getting worse. We have seen that children with ARFID may struggle in a variety of different ways and also that children with a broad range of abilities and personal and medical histories can develop avoidance and restriction of food intake. This chapter aims to set out of some of the basic principles that you can apply as a parent or primary carer; not all of these may be relevant to your situation, but hopefully some of them will be. This is the first of the two *care* chapters in the book.

In our discussion on *causes* (Chapter 3: Why does someone develop ARFID?) the statement was made that it is rarely helpful to get into a way of thinking along the lines of fault, blame or regret. Such feelings tend to paralyse situations rather than help them change. Their presence is not usually in your best interests or the best interests of your child. If you think your partner or someone else is at fault, your energy will probably go into arguing with them. If you think you are to blame for your child's eating difficulties, you will most likely be undermining your own confidence in your parenting abilities, which can lead to feelings of hopelessness and helplessness. If you dwell on regrets, wishing certain things had not happened, or giving yourself a hard time because they did, that does nothing to change the impact of those events. Very importantly, if you think in terms of fault, blame, and regret, you may well think that other people share these thoughts. This can be extremely unhelpful. If you assume that others blame you, you are much more likely to become defensive, to refuse offers of help or to be reluctant try things someone else has suggested. So, how best to take positive steps to support your child?

One thing that can be helpful in trying to change any situation, whether you are someone with a problem to change, a parent, or a professional, is to work through what has become known as 'the 5-step model' (Bryant-Waugh 2006). This is also sometimes referred to as 'the underwear sequence', which requires some explanation! The five steps that make up this sequence are illustrated in Figure 5.1.

As you will see, the five steps are named Explore, Understand, Accept, Challenge, Change. They represent a sequence of tasks that can be helpful to work through in order, in attempting to change things in a positive direction. As it is not always easy to remember sequences, people often make up rhymes or memorable phrases to help with recall. Such memory aids are called 'mnemonics'; these are essentially tools to help us remember information. For example, you may be familiar with the mnemonic sometimes used to help children learn how to spell 'because': Big

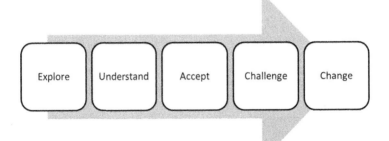

Figure 5.1 The 5-step model towards change

Elephants Can't Always Understand Small Elephants. Another well-known example is the acronym FAST, which can help us remember what to do if you suspect someone is having a stroke – to check their Face, Arms, Speech and if you notice that any of these have been affected, it is Time to make the call to emergency services. In the case of the 5-step model, one mnemonic to remember the sequence of the steps is: Exotic Underwear Always Causes Chaos. The first letters of each word correspond with the first letter of each step – Explore, Understand, Accept, Challenge, Change. The idea of any mnemonic is that it should be memorable! You may well come up with one you think more suitable, but this is the reason the 5-step model is known to some as the 'underwear sequence'.

Let's explore the five steps in a bit more detail to understand why working through each in turn is so important. One of the things that often happens, when people try to change their own or someone else's behaviour, is that once the problem has been identified, they tend to come straight in at the 'challenge' stage hoping that this will lead to change. They might say, OK, this is the problem that we/I need to get rid of, without having considered why it might be there in the first place and what might be keeping it going. This might sometimes work, but in the majority of cases it is unlikely to be effective without a great deal of determination. The reason for this is that most behaviours that persist have some kind of positive function. If I habitually bite my nails, even though I may not like how my hands look as a consequence, I may keep doing it when I am nervous or anxious, because it gives me something to do at these times and helps me tolerate unpleasant feelings. If I am to stop doing it, I need to develop an awareness of when I do it and why, and think about other strategies that I might be able to use. Coming in directly to challenge behaviour without understanding it better may lead to attempts to change it failing. In turn, this can leave people feeling demoralised or losing hope in ever being able to be successful. Most human behaviour makes sense to the person engaging in it. It often serves a purpose or has a function that provides some positive feedback. If you simply try to stop a behaviour that is serving some kind of positive function, without considering the impact of taking it away and addressing this, it is understandable that attempts to do so may not be successful. We know that taking a step back to *explore* the background to the behaviour in order to arrive at a better understanding of it is often essential to successful behavioural change. To *understand* a behaviour is much more than just recognising that a problem exists (and getting cross or frustrated about it); why has it developed and what function does it serve? Once we have a better understanding of the existence of the problem behaviour, we then need to *accept* that – at present – this is how things are. No fault, no blame, no regret. It just is that way now. This allows us to consider whether we want to change it, to *challenge* to status quo. What will be the consequences of making changes? What are the advantages and disadvantages? Once we have been all through this, and taken account of things as fully as we can, then we can begin the process of *change* with a much better chance of success.

Let's consider these steps in relation to a child with avoidance and restriction of food intake. We will go through each in turn. Table 5.1 captures some of the things covered in the sections below and may be useful to refer back to.

Explore

To help you explore your child's eating behaviour in terms of exactly what type of difficulties they are experiencing, it might be helpful to refer back to the section on *characteristics* (Chapter 1: What is ARFID?). You might want to check the answers to a few key questions, and make a note of your impressions:

1 If avoidance or restriction of food intake is present, is this in relation to the overall amount eaten (i.e. the overall calorie intake), in relation to the range of foods eaten (i.e. the overall nutritional adequacy of the intake), or both of these?

   This question is important as it can help to determine whether it is most appropriate for your child to try to increase portion sizes or the number of times they eat during the day, or whether they need to try to introduce new foods and/or a multi-vitamin and mineral supplement. In some cases, you

Table 5.1 Applying the 5-step model to ARFID

Explore	Understand	Accept	Challenge	Change
Characteristics	Correlates and Causes	Making Sense	Consequences	Care
Avoidance or restriction: • In terms of amount (calories)? • In terms of range (nutrients)? **Duration of difficulties?** • Longstanding or more recent? **On supplements?** • What supplement? • How much? • How given (oral or tube)? • When given? **Where is problem obvious?** • At home? • At school? • With relatives? • With friends? • When out?	**What are main drivers of avoidance/restriction?** • Low interest? • Sensory sensitivities? • Concern about consequences? **Why might these be present?** • Disrupted appetite regulation (e.g. due to tube feeding)? • Reduced or low desire (due to mood, stress, over-arousal, concentration difficulties, persistent undereating)? • Oral-motor difficulties? • Concurrent illness/condition? • Side effects of medication?	**Accepting** that your child is unlikely to be deliberately wilful, naughty or behaving in an irrational way **Accepting** that your child's eating behaviour is most likely related to normal fight, flight or avoidance responses **Understanding** why these responses might be present **Accepting** that this is just how things currently are without undue feelings of guilt or blame **Understanding** that this is not how things need to stay for ever	**What needs to be changed?** • Impact on weight/growth/development? • Improving nutrition? • Dependence on supplements or tube feeds? • Impact on family life and arrangements around eating? • Mealtime arguments and stress • Impact on learning and ability to participate in normal age appropriate activities? • Social isolation and struggles eating with others or when out • Impact on other family members • Other family members' understanding?	**Setting about making changes, by:** • Following the 5-step model sequence • Writing things down to take with you to appointments • Minimising confrontation and stress at the table • Being realistic about expectations • Being clear and consistent • Helping your child to take risks with their eating

Check not related to:

- Weight/shape related avoidance
- Other explanatory condition/situation

What is current risk?

- High, medium, low?

Is risk related to?

- Weight/growth/development?
- Nutritional status?
- Impact on child's psychological wellbeing and development?
- Impact on the family?

- Being a supertaster/supersenser?
- Feelings of disgust?
- Fear related to previous negative experiences?
- Worries picked up from someone?
- Temperamental anxiety

Is your child in a higher risk group?

- Has ASD or ADHD?
- Has learning disability?
- Has a complex medical history with interruptions to feeding?
- Is temperamentally cautious, rigid, stubborn?
- From a family with a history of restricted eating?

Having **explored** things and moved to a position of **understanding** your child's eating behaviour as a logical response under the circumstances and **accepting** this, being ready to move to a position to think about what could be different and how this can be achieved, to **challenge** the status quo and move towards **change**

What is keeping things going?

- Habit?
- Positive consequences for child?
- Fixed beliefs, attitudes, thoughts?

Do the adults agree about wanting to make changes and ready to work together?

What might the barriers be to making progress?

Is your child motivated to make changes?

- If not why do you think this is?

- Appreciating even small steps
- Explaining clearly to family and friends
- Working alongside professionals as appropriate
- Sharing the load
- Dealing with any feelings of blame and guilt

may need to try to support your child to do both. This is also an important question in relation to considering how serious you think the problem is. Is it obviously affecting their weight or growth? Do they seem pale or tired all the time because of poor diet? If in doubt, it is best to seek medical advice.

2   How long have the eating difficulties been going on? Is this a longstanding problem and likely to have become quite a habit? Has your child eaten better in the past? Do the difficulties have a more recent onset, perhaps related to a bad experience?

These questions are important as they can help you with your expectations of change. If your child has never eaten like their peers, it may take longer to be able to manage a wide range of foods or they may initially struggle with eating more. However, if your child has previously eaten a wider range or a greater quantity of food, in principle they should be able to go back to do doing so if all the steps in the 5-step model are worked through in turn.

3   Is your child on food supplements? If so which supplements and how much are they having? Does your child take them via a tube or do they take them by mouth? When are these given?

These questions are important as they help you think about opening up areas for possible change. If your child is being tube fed, are you still offering food in the normal way? Tube feeding can leave children feeling quite full, so is there any scope to adjust the timing of the tube feeds to allow them to feel hungrier at any time in the day? If you are giving a multivitamin and mineral supplement, are you giving one that contains the things that seem to be missing from their diet? Have you tried to get them to take a hard or a chewy tablet but they have refused this? What about a liquid version? It can be very helpful to write down exactly what supplements your child is having and when these are given if you attend an appointment with a doctor or a dietitian. They will be able to advise you if anything is missing or any changes can be made to type of supplement, timing, and how these are administered.

4   Is your child's eating more or less the same wherever they are or whoever they are with? What about at school, or when with relatives or friends? If you go out as a family is your child's eating better, worse or the same?

This is important to explore as it might give an idea of where efforts to make changes might first be directed. For example, if your child tends to eat better with their grandmother, then that might be the best place to start to introduce something new, however much you might prefer to do this at home. Making it as likely as possible that your child might succeed is very important, and once something has been changed or something new introduced, then they are more likely to be able to work on doing this at home. Many children seem to eat a bit better at school, although some may struggle even more in this environment. We know that children often behave very differently at school to how they behave at home and that parents can experience this as frustrating! Many children are more likely to conform and do as they are told at school and again this might mean this is the environment to begin to work on small changes which can then later be practised in different environments, including home. It is important to place any feelings of disappointment to one side, if home is where the biggest struggles are, and to really try to identify where your child's eating seems slightly easier (if this is the case – some children do not waver at all in their eating habits irrespective of where they are). Some children seem to eat better when travelling in a car or a train, or when on a beach or outside (often due to the sensation of movement and visual stimulation dampening sensory overload from food), so be prepared to be creative. The point is to explore if there are any situations where you might be in with a better chance to help your child make changes.

5   Is the restriction or avoidance of food to do with your child being worried about being too big or too heavy? Are they cutting down on the amount they eat, or only choosing certain foods because they think it will help them lose weight? Is there some other clear reason why your child's intake is limited, such as copying other members of the family going on a

diet? Or are you struggling to provide enough food for your child?

These questions are important because as we have seen, if the main reason for avoiding food or restricting intake is to do with significant worries about weight and shape, your child may be engaging in dieting behaviour, or may be developing signs of an eating disorder such as anorexia nervosa or bulimia nervosa. It is rarely advisable for children to go on very low calorie diets. Children need to grow and develop and at most, if the child is overweight, the aim is generally to halt weight gain rather than achieve drastic weight loss. In people with ARFID, whatever age they are, the avoidance and restriction is not driven by concerns about weight and shape. It is also not related to there simply not being enough food.

6   Do you think there might be another reason that could explain why your child may be avoiding or restricting their food intake? Are they very constipated or do they have diarrhoea? Do they have any persistent or unusual stomach pains? Are they vomiting? Do they have other symptoms that might suggest something else might be going on, like a rash, or joint pains, or regular mouth ulcers?

These questions are important as there are lots of reasons that children's food intake may be limited or may diminish. If you notice anything out of the ordinary that is giving you cause for concern, it is usually best to visit your family doctor or speak to someone who may be able to provide advice.

7   Is your child's eating having a negative impact on their ability to participate in age-appropriate activities? Is it impairing their day-to-day functioning? What about the impact on yourself and on other members of the family?

These questions are important in determining the extent of the impact of your child's eating difficulties in terms of their social and emotional functioning as well as the impact the situation may be having on others. Children and young people are learning all the time to manage their emotions and to interact with others; these aspects of normal development are very important. When children miss out, for whatever reason, they may fall behind their peers which can leave them feeling isolated. Promoting participation in age-appropriate activities and having expectations of children that are appropriate for their stage of development is an important aspect of positive parenting. Most children need to learn how to function in society and ultimately to become independent from their parents in this respect. If your child's eating difficulties are beginning to hold them back, attention to helping them back on track in terms of social and emotional development may be needed. Clearly children will have different levels of potential in this respect; for example, children with severe autism or those with learning disabilities may be missing out just as much in their own way due to limitations caused by eating difficulties.

Many parents of children with ARFID report feeling quite low or overwhelmed with worries at times. Some may experience feelings of failure or inadequacy. After all, feeding your child is a fundamental aspect of effective parenting. It is unsurprising that things can seem very difficult and we know that some parents really struggle with these negative feelings, to the extent that they may suffer from episodes of depression or anxiety. If you feel you have symptoms of these problems, including sleep disruption, loss of appetite, mood disturbance, withdrawal, frequent tearfulness, or loss of pleasure in most things, do make sure you seek appropriate advice and support.

Parents also report that the eating behaviour of the child who is avoiding or restricting their food intake can adversely affect brothers and sisters or others in the family. Siblings may copy refusal behaviours leaving some parents unsure how best to manage. Many families try to have mealtime and eating rules that apply to everyone, so that it can feel difficult to justify why one child can have the same foods every day, some of which parents may limit for their other children. Some parents end up making different meals for each child because siblings have rejected the family meal on the basis that the child with ARFID tends to get their preferred food. Balancing being fair and making exceptions can be difficult. However, if your child does have ARFID, as we have seen, this is not something they will have chosen and is not helpfully considered as bad behaviour or naughtiness. It is a recognised condition and in the same way you would make different arrangements for a child with a food allergy, it might be necessary to be clear about why things are different, at least at present.

Making a note of the answers to the above questions can help you capture your views of the characteristics and impact of your child's difficulties. This information will be very important if you seek further advice and support and can be extremely helpful for the clinicians whom you see. Your experiences and knowledge of changes in your child and your family are not held by anyone else. You are the expert in this respect.

Understand

This step is about trying to make sense of things, to arrive at an understanding why your child might be avoiding or restricting their intake. Is it primarily due to low interest in food and eating, sensory based avoidance or concern about aversive consequences of eating? Or do you recognise a combination of these things? Is your child expressing fear or disgust or both? Why might these things be present? We have seen in Chapters 2 and 3 when we discussed *correlates* and *causes* that some children may be more inclined to develop ARFID or fall into a higher risk group, due to their temperament, to co-occurring conditions, or because of things that they may have experienced. Previous difficult experiences with food or eating may be continuing to cause your child worry and this may contribute to ongoing refusal or resistance. It is often worth sitting down and thinking through everything you think might have contributed. Perhaps it might be helpful to re-read Chapters 2 and 3. You could make a note of things you think could be relevant to try to put them together to arrive at a clearer understanding of why you might be facing the struggles you currently experience in encouraging your child to eat adequately. Writing it down like this can also be helpful to take with you if you seek medical or other professional advice.

Accept

Accepting that this is how things are at present does not mean you have to be complacent about it. It is often appropriate to worry about a child who isn't eating well! It is more about a point at which you bring things together and move to a position of thinking, I might understand this a bit better now, before moving on to consider how best to work on change. It might be helpful to think of it as the swing of a pendulum – when the pendulum is at the maximum height of its swing trajectory, it is charged with momentum for the downward fall. The *explore* and *understand* steps can be thought of as the upward swing to this point, with the still point at the top being the *accept* stage, before sweeping back down through *challenge* to ultimately arrive at *change*, with the desired goals of change being the equilibrium point at the base. Exploring, understanding and then accepting the situation for what it is can help with gathering momentum in the form of improved clarity of direction and purpose, and feeling more positive about being able to make changes.

Challenge

During this fourth step in the process of addressing current difficulties, the main questions are whether things have to stay this way and whether there is real potential for change. The main tasks here include thinking through the detail of what needs changing most, exploring how this might be achieved, asking how realistic this is, and considering what the impact, positive as well as negative, of making changes might be. Here, it can be helpful to think about the *consequences* of your child's current eating difficulties, as broadly as possible, and again make a list of these. It might be useful to re-read Chapter 4 (What are the consequences of ARFID?) at this point. This can assist in helping you decide what seems most important to try to improve. There will often be multiple areas of impact and it will be difficult to tackle all at once. Being able to break things down and deciding to work on specific areas can feel less overwhelming and much more do-able.

Remember that behaviour often serves a positive function. One consequence of this is that if you take it away or change it, replacement behaviours may pop up to fill the gap it left, if the reason for engaging in the behaviour in the first place remains unchanged. For example, let's imagine a child who is extremely anxious and whose eating difficulties were triggered by hearing about a group of people suffering from severe food poisoning in a restaurant. If that child is successfully helped back to their previous more normal eating behaviour without the underlying generalised anxiety being addressed, it is quite likely that other problematic behaviours may develop in the future. These may be nothing to do with eating, for example, the same child might start refusing to leave the house because of an incident of violence on the local streets. In the *challenge* stage, it can be helpful to think about the impact of making changes in this way too. Would it leave a gap? By the end of this step you should hopefully feel much clearer about what you feel needs to be changed and why, what the barriers might be, and what might help. Ideally, you will feel ready and positive about proceeding to the very important step of working on *change*.

Change

Formal treatment for ARFID will be discussed in the next chapter (Chapter 6: What is the best treatment for ARFID?). You will be able to read about the main strategies known to be helpful in managing avoidant and restrictive eating behaviours in children and young people; hopefully some of these will feel relevant to your own situation.

There are in addition a few areas that you can attend to alongside. It is important to try, as far as possible, to adhere to some key principles in the process of working towards change. These include:

- keeping worries in perspective
- remaining consistent in how you are managing and supporting your child's eating
- remembering to use what you know about good parenting

- being clear and unapologetic about any adjustments or accommodations that may be needed whilst you are working with your child on making changes
- looking after yourself.

Keeping worries in perspective

It is very important to keep worries and concerns in perspective throughout the process of making change. This can often be easier said than done! Table 5.2 represents a reminder of the four key areas of risk we have already discussed. If the answer to these questions is 'yes', then certainly, continued concerted efforts are required to make change happen. If the answer is 'no', or these things are present to a lesser extent, then there is generally time to work on things at the appropriate pace for your child. Over-worrying and existing with high levels of day-to-day stress about a situation are not likely to benefit anyone. They are likely to increase your own distress and may leave you feeling more frustrated, impatient, and upset than is warranted for the situation. If there are 'yes' answers to the questions in Table 5.2, it is probably time to seek help if you haven't already done so!

Remaining consistent in how you are managing and supporting your child's eating

Consistency is vital in helping children to change their behaviour. They will need you to do exactly what you say you are going to do. They will need to know what is expected of them and they will need you not to change your mind at the last minute. They will also need all the adults involved in their care or in their lives to be giving a similar message as far as possible. Let's look at an example. If you have agreed to try something new with your child, say a potato which they are expecting to try alongside their familiar slice of chicken, then on that occasion stick with the potato, even if it seems to be eaten without difficulty. The

Table 5.2 Key areas of risk in relation to ARFID in children and young people

Weight, growth and physical development	Nutritional adequacy of diet
• Has your child stopped growing as expected because they are not eating adequately? • Is your child losing weight because they are not taking in enough calories? • Has pubertal development been put on hold because of the eating difficulties?	• Does your child have clear signs or symptoms of a nutritional deficiency because of a poor diet? • Are any of the major food groups (proteins, carbohydrates and starchy foods, fruit/vegetables, dairy/dairy alternatives, oils and spreads) missing from their diet that is not supplemented for in any way?
Impact on child's social and emotional development	Impact on family functioning?
• Is your child suffering from distress related to their eating behaviour? • Is your child missing out on key activities with peers they might otherwise be expected to take part in because of limitations imposed by their eating habits? • Is your child struggling to attend or to keep up at school because of their eating difficulties?	• Are there frequent rows and arguments because of the child's eating? • Is anyone in the family experiencing significant mood changes or developing challenging behaviour as a consequence of the child's eating difficulties? • Is family life severely restricted (e.g. unable to go on holiday, eat out, stay with relatives) because of limitations imposed by the child's eating habits?

temptation is to say something like, 'well, that was too easy so you need to try a carrot as well!' A better approach would be to say something like, 'Well done! That was fantastic work!' adding 'Perhaps we can try something different next time?' If you push beyond what has been agreed because it seemed too easy, you run the risk of not recognising the child's effort at trying something new. Your child may become demoralised and unsure where the boundaries of your expectations lie. You also run the risk of losing your child's trust and their willingness to engage in trying things. Your job is to support and encourage your child to feel safe enough to take risks. Consistency is also important between parents and other individuals who may be present at or supervising mealtimes. Children with ARFID generally manage much better with predictability and prior knowledge about expectations. This doesn't mean the goal posts can't be changed, just that the child needs to know where they are at any one time, and that they are in the same place irrespective of which parent or carer might be with them. In the same way, it is important to be consistent about what is being worked on. Is it overall amount eaten? Adding new foods into their diet? Helping them move away from tube feeding? Working on socially useful foods? It can be confusing for children if there are sudden changes to the plan. These can backfire as what might seem like an easy and logical next step might be experienced by the child as significantly difficult and therefore resisted.

In children with low interest in food and eating, consistency will be required in the process of gradually working on a more regular pattern of eating, or increasing portion sizes (see further Chapter 7). A planned period of increasing expectation with appropriate support, clearly communicated to the child, is more likely to be effective than random bursts of effort followed by periods with little attention to working to change the child's eating. Maintaining consistency can require parents to consciously work at keeping their motivation to support their child to make changes high. The pace of change can be slow, and when daily effort is also needed from parents, it is not difficult to see why people might get tired, bored or frustrated with the process and decide to take a break. Taking breaks is fine, as long as they are planned and predictable and as long as they have a clearly stated purpose or reason (e.g. to consolidate gains made). The key with consistency is to help your child feel safer with the whole process. They usually have enough to feel unsafe about already in relation to changes to their eating behaviour.

Consistency in managing family mealtimes can also be important. Generally, the advice given is to try to limit arguments and stress at the table. Here again the child needs to know what will be expected of them in terms of eating and what support they might get from you with this. It is best to be clear about this before the meal starts. If the child then struggles, complains loudly, refuses, shouts, or engages in disruptive behaviour, it is best to avoid a battle there and then, but return to what made it so difficult, away from the table. Many parents report that advice to 'back off' and allow the child to initiate interest has been very helpful in working towards change. If children feel pressured and wary of what might be sprung upon them every time they sit down for a meal, it seems reasonable that their defences, in the form of sticking rigidly to what they know, might be raised. There are no hard and fast rules about the detailed content of plans and expectations, but the principle of being consistent once these have been decided is vital.

Remembering to use what you know about good parenting

Most parents naturally have access to positive parenting skills. We are genetically wired to care for our young, as are almost all mammals. Some parents, for example, those who have specific and severe mental health problems, histories of complex trauma or abuse, or significant learning disabilities, may be impaired in their capacity to exercise their parental instincts, but generally we are protective and nurturing towards our offspring. Of course that goes for parents of children with ARFID too! We have seen how having a child with eating difficulties can cause some parents to doubt their parenting abilities. In families where the child with ARFID has siblings who eat normally, this is perhaps curious, but not uncommon. To an outsider, the parents are clearly competent as their other children are fine. Some parents have a number of children with difficulties. This is usually nothing to do with their parenting, but often more to do with genetic loading increasing the likelihood that their offspring will have specific conditions. In this chapter on what you can do if your child has ARFID, it might be helpful to review a couple of strategies that most people reading this will be very well aware of, but might have lost sight of in their attempts to help their child.

First and foremost, it is important to engender trust in the relationship with your child. Children who grow up in the context of secure, trusting relationships have been shown to be able to form positive, loving, social relationships as adults. Your child needs to be able to trust you, as when they are young, you are the fixed point they will return to as they negotiate the challenges of growing up. Sometimes parents who are desperately worried about their child's eating report that they 'sneak' things into their child's preferred foods to try to get some 'goodness' in. Common examples include adding some vegetables into something already eaten, or putting drops into yoghurt, without the child knowing. This is not uncommon for many parents to do when their children are very young, or during weaning. However, in children with ARFID, the result can be that the child detects even a small amount of something added (remember the child with ARFID may be a super-taster or be able to detect even very small changes in texture) and then refuses to eat the preferred food completely as they have lost trust that it is an OK thing to eat. They may also lose trust in you and in some cases refuse to eat anything other than packaged food of certain brands, insisting on opening the packet themselves. Trust relies on good communication, as well as the consistency and predictability described above. If you are introducing new things, it may be best to be clear about it and to allow your child to continue to enjoy their 'safe' foods.

Another aspect of good parenting that mostly comes naturally, is praising a child when they do something you like or want them to do. Think of your baby's first smile. You probably didn't ignore it! Most parents will smile back and make encouraging noises. Children learn in this way that they get positive attention, which includes praise, when they do something we like, which in turn encourages them to do it again. In children with ARFID, it is really important to positively acknowledge the child's effort when this is appropriate and give praise when praise is due, even if what has been achieved seems tiny. It is very easy to unintentionally reinforce negative behaviour, by getting cross or frustrated, particularly if any positive behaviours are not acknowledged at all because they don't seem much.

We are also programmed to be protective of our young; some of us are more so than others! Children need parental support in being able to move away from the complete dependence of babyhood, through childhood and adolescence to adulthood. One constructive way that parents of children with ARFID can be protective is to help them understand their difficulties better, develop ways of managing difficult or unexpected situations involving food, and helping them to explain their intention not to eat something to others. It is often best to help children to use everyday, truthful language that makes clear, for example, that at present they don't eat some foods. Primary school aged children are usually used to some peers having dietary exclusions due to allergies or specific medical conditions. Your child does not need to explain the full detail; they just need to be able to manage situations where they might be faced with foods they feel unable to eat. It is more important that they feel confident to take part in such situations, rather than avoid them in case someone mentions food.

Being clear and unapologetic about any adjustments or accommodations that may be needed whilst you are working with your child on making changes

Just as your child needs to be equipped with the language to manage social situations involving food, it is also helpful for parents to be able to explain the situation to others as needed without being apologetic, feeling shame or any sense of inadequacy. It can be helpful to explain that your child has a condition that is currently being treated, or that you are all working to resolve, but at present this brings certain constraints, limitations or requirements with it. It is important to be comfortable explaining the situation without being overly defensive. It can feel very isolating having a child with ARFID and so this may not be easy. Reminding yourself of what you know about ARFID and being clear and concise in your explanations are strategies worth developing. This is likely to include communication with your child's school if this is needed. It can be helpful to anticipate that understanding of

ARFID may be limited and to be as matter of fact and as unapologetic as you can. If understanding is better than you thought, so much the better, but if it seems as if the school needs some persuading that the problem is genuine, then you will be better prepared for that. You and your child would be unlikely to choose to be in this situation so you don't need to apologise for it. It may be that your child might benefit from some special accommodations at school, such as being placed in a less busy part of the dining area, being allowed to access a snack during the morning, or having permission to bring certain foods into school despite these generally not being permitted in the interests of promoting 'healthy eating'. It is always best to try to have a calm, friendly discussion with relevant school staff about what might help. Be prepared to listen to suggestions they might have, as it is very common for children to behave differently at school, and their suggestions may be worth a try. Be ready to offer to provide more information about ARFID in general and to explain that this is something you are working to address. If special arrangements are agreed, it is usually helpful to set a time when these will be reviewed. After half a term or so, it may be possible to take a next step in supporting your child to manage eating with peers; this is after all an important aspect of their social development. Here again, clarity in relation to the plan and consistency between adults are also likely to be of most benefit to your child.

Looking after yourself

Last and by no means least, one further thing you can do to optimise the care of your child, is to make sure you look after yourself. You will be a much more effective parent if you do not set yourself up to fail but focus on maintaining your own confidence and ability to function from one day to the next. Check your expectations of your child's ability to change; are they realistic? Do you feel prepared for challenges that may lie ahead? If your child becomes distressed, will you be able to remain consistent? Do you understand how what you are proposing to do might help your child, or does it feel wrong? If the latter, then take time to try to understand the rationale, as doing something you do not feel is in your child's best interests is likely to result in you feeling stressed and unhappy, and increases the chance of confusing your child. Are you experiencing feelings of blame or guilt? If so, you may need to work on this. Perhaps discuss the situation with someone close to you whom you trust. If you have relatives who don't hold back in expressing views that if your child had been brought up by them there wouldn't be problems, do not forget what you know. They probably do not know much about ARFID and may misunderstand the difficulties you and your child are facing. Do not spend too much time with people who make you feel miserable and inadequate. Be aware of the tendency for guilt and self-blame to creep back in, especially if progress is slow. Try to keep it in check. You will need to consider carefully how you feel about the situation and take responsibility for trying to make sure you are in as good a frame of mind as possible so that you can support your child. You might need to develop a thicker skin.

Another aspect of looking after yourself is allowing others to share the load. If it is possible, take some time out; this does not have to be long, even one mealtime every now and then might feel like a break. If you have a partner, discuss with them how all your children's needs can best be met whilst working on improving the child with ARFID's eating and how these tasks can be divided. If you don't have a partner, see if relatives or friends can help out a bit. Everyone needs a bit of time off in order to return to a task with renewed energy.

In this chapter we have discussed some of the things it may be helpful for you to focus on and to do in the process of helping your child. In the next chapter we will look in more detail at specific treatment approaches for ARFID.

Chapter 6

What is the best treatment for ARFID?

This is the second of the *care* chapters. It includes what is known about treatment for ARFID; which approaches might be appropriate for different aspects of the condition; how to decide the best way to proceed for any one individual; and what you and your child might be offered if you attend a clinic. In order to provide a logical structure to the chapter, we will begin first by discussing the importance of thorough assessment by clinicians with appropriate skills and knowledge. We will then move to the model for evidence-based practice, referred to in the Introduction, based on three key principles and apply these to ARFID.

Careful, detailed assessment is often the key to identifying the best treatment for your child. Much of what we have already considered in this book should ideally be covered at the assessment stage. The first two columns of Table 5.1 in Chapter 5 capture some of the questions that are helpfully included in a good assessment. As we have seen, the task is to explore the background and detail of current difficulties and to try to arrive at a means of understanding why your child might be struggling with their eating. Much of the material in Chapter 1 (What is ARFID?) as well as Chapters 2 and 3 (Who can develop ARFID? and Why does someone develop ARFID?), which cover *characteristics, correlates* and *causes* respectively, needs to be covered. With this information we can begin to construct a picture of where the major difficulties lie that seem to be keeping the problem going. Exactly what is holding your child back? If we can identify this, it already becomes somewhat clearer what support might be needed and where it might be possible to achieve some change. A diagnosis of ARFID alone actually tells us very little about how best to approach treatment, making the importance of this first assessment stage an integral part of good treatment planning.

As well as trying to make sense of things and being able to accept that the current situation, although difficult, is unlikely to be any one person's fault and is unlikely to be impossible to change, good treatment planning also includes an assessment of risk. This is important as clearly if risk is high in relation to one or more aspects of your child's situation, this will need attention in the first instance. The material covered in Chapter 4 (What are the consequences of ARFID?), and set out in the fourth column of Table 5.1, points to the sort of things that are helpfully included in this part of the assessment. Risk can be present in relation to the child's physical state, their mental health and emotional well-being, their overall development, or all of these things. Risk can also be related to your own mental health and emotional well-being, the child's siblings, and family life. Sometimes children's behaviour can become very challenging, directed at themselves or towards others, and sometimes family members can become so frustrated or distressed by the scale and intensity of eating difficulties, that the child may be at risk of harm. If significant risk is identified in any of these areas, this will by necessity form an early focus for treatment.

Because ARFID is a disturbance in eating behaviour that can significantly impair both physical health and day-to-day psychological, social, and educational functioning, and because avoidance and restriction of food intake can have multiple causes, the kind of detailed assessment described above will usually involve different types of clinicians. Current consensus is that although ARFID may be screened for and identified as a possible diagnosis by one well-informed clinician, comprehensive assessment, including risk assessment, generally requires multi-disciplinary input. This is also important to make sure other conditions that might be causing the eating difficulties are not missed. It may be that treatment can be delivered by one type of clinician, but commonly, in this respect too, representatives with different professional backgrounds and training are involved. Those most likely to provide input besides primary care doctors are paediatricians, psychologists, dietitians, nurses, speech and language therapists, and occupational therapists. Other professionals that may be involved are family therapists, social workers, psychiatrists, play workers, and specialist doctors such as gastroenterologists. In children with learning disabilities, severe autism, or other specific needs requiring special education provision, teachers and class-room assistants may also form part of the treatment team. Of course the child's parents or carers form the core of the treating team; they have the most knowledge about the child and their own family context.

Following assessment therefore, it should be possible to move to the 'challenge' and 'change' steps on the 5-step model described in Chapter 5. Considering what needs to be changed and ensuring everyone is on the same page in terms of what is required, or as close to it as possible, is very important in terms of treatment planning. As long as any immediate risk is managed, it is extre-mely important that the child's primary caregivers are ready and willing to work with each other and with the treating team to implement consistent strategies. This means that any differences in view or opinion may need to be ironed out or set aside and that tasks are clear. At the start of treatment children may not be at all interested in making changes; in fact they may be positively fear-ful or resistant. Most parents would agree that the process of treating ARFID is often far from easy, with moments of doubt, particularly in the face of a child's distress. Under such circum-stances, being clear what you are doing and why, and being able to seek support from or offer support to a partner, co-parent, or other caregiver can make a huge difference. If your child has ARFID, eating is difficult for them. Changing that is likely to require persistence, consistency, and conviction. Clinicians may refer to such things as 'engagement' and 'motivation'; they will often want to assess the extent to which those involved are actively ready and willing to work on the difficulties, and how keen they are to make changes. Sometimes some work is needed to make sure things are as solidly set up as possible in terms of everyone being ready and willing to work together. Generally this is time well spent as this can form the bedrock for treatment approaches to have the highest chance of working. Perhaps an analogy for gardeners is the knowledge that taking time to thoroughly dig over and weed a flower bed before planting out tiny seedlings will allow a greater chance that they will thrive, than if they are competing with more robust opportunistic plants from the start.

Having discussed assessment, members of the treating team, and basic preparations for getting started, we now need to turn our attention to specific components of treatment. In order to organise the material to be covered, we will use the three pillared model of evidence-based practice (Sackett et al. 1996; Sackett et al. 2000). This is now a widely adopted approach in health-care, but one which deserves a little explanation. In most countries with organised health-care services supported by public funds, there is a clear expectation that clinical practitioners will provide interventions or deliver treatments that are based on evidence that they are safe, appropriate or effective. This is not perhaps as self-evident as you may think. It is still not uncommon that practitioners may offer treatments that are not supported by any formal research demonstrating that they are particularly helpful. The history of medicine is littered with examples of now discontinued practices that turned out to actually make patients worse. Although this is now thankfully much rarer, it is of course important that we know as far as possible that what we are doing is not going to cause harm. This has long been a central tenet of medicine; the first promise of anyone becoming a doctor is 'first, do no harm', dating back to the time of Hippocrates in ancient Greece. Nowadays, our ability to capture and acquire information is of course unrecognisably different, but we do still have gaps in our knowledge. Sometimes we are unaware of things, sometimes we have not asked the right questions in our research, and sometimes the studies have simply not been carried out. In terms of research findings that can be used to inform clinical practice, information obtained through well designed studies is crucial. If a study is poorly designed or not properly carried out, it is impossible to make sense of the results. One type of study design in particular, the 'randomised controlled trial' is generally considered the gold standard. This design removes as far as possible anything that might muddle the results and interfere with being able to report clearly and accurately on the specific effects and outcomes of any one treatment or other type of intervention. These results can then be used to guide evidence-based practice. However, randomised controlled treatment trials are often expensive to run, difficult to carry out, and in some cases simply do not exist to answer all the questions we may have about the best treatments for different conditions.

How then should responsible clinicians proceed? This is where the three pillar model comes in. This proposes that evidence-based practice should be supported by three equally important pillars of evidence. The first of these is represented by information obtained through clinically relevant, well conducted, well designed research studies, preferably of the standard of a randomised controlled trial. The second pillar is represented by accumulated clinical expertise; what is known from experience of treating large numbers of people with specific conditions about what works and what doesn't work. This second pillar is in part informed by the clinician's training, but also by the expertise they have acquired and the skills they have developed. The third pillar is represented by patient values and preferences. We know that what the patient brings to any health-care encounter, in terms of their expectations, their wishes, things that are important to them, their concerns and their past experiences, are important to the outcome of that encounter. The three pillar model of evidence-based practice is appealing because it stresses the importance of attending to these patient values, just as much as attending to what the clinician knows, and what research evidence shows. In this model good evidence-based practice arises from an integration of these three components.

We will proceed with discussing best treatment for ARFID using this model. Starting first with patient values, moving on to clinical expertise, and finishing with best research evidence. In the case of ARFID in children, 'patient values' includes the values, hopes, expectations, and experiences of parents or primary caregivers. Parents act on behalf of their children in addressing their healthcare needs, exercising their parental rights and responsibilities. If we are to attend to patient values in treatment, we need to take full account of what is causing concern, and what the impact of the current difficulties is for those directly affected.

Parents attending our clinic have been quite consistent about aspects of their child's eating that concern them most. They include:

- the quantity of food the child eats
- the variety of food the child eats
- the child's dependence on tube-feeding or supplements
- the child's lack of willingness to try new foods
- the inability to eat any solid food
- the quality of the child's diet
- problems with chewing and swallowing
- the child's fear of food
- mealtime behaviour
- lack of interest in food/low appetite
- how long the child takes to eat

These all seem very understandable concerns. You may share some of them with regard to your own child. It makes sense that treatment should address such concerns if they exist. It may be that the clinician identifies other areas of risk, for example in relation to the child's physical state that the parents may not have considered. In such cases treatment will need to combine both areas of concern to provide optimal treatment.

Another aspect of patient values that clinicians need to take account of in treatment planning, is the impact the child's eating difficulties are reported to be having on both the child and the family. This can be difficult to determine from the specific clinical detail of the ARFID presentation alone and relies on listening to the family. Again, parents attending our clinic tended to be quite consistent about key areas that they feel are adversely affected by the child's eating difficulties. They include:

- impairment to the child's social life
- faltering growth, lack of weight gain or losing weight
- impairment to general health
- the child's intake of vitamins and minerals in their diet
- negative effects on the child's mood
- exacerbating other existing medical conditions

- making family mealtimes very difficult
- reducing the child's stamina

The three pillar model of evidence-based practice supports the need to take such things into account and to work in a way that fits with the family's needs and preferences to achieve meaningful changes. Very often parents might say that they have simply been told that their child is growing and their weight is fine and so there is nothing to worry about. If you have a child you struggle with on a daily basis to ensure they get enough to keep them going, you are going to have a different view of things! Good patient-centred care, which is widely regarded as 'best treatment', therefore involves clinicians listening carefully and discussing priorities with you to achieve an agreed way forward. It involves attending to the child's and the family's engagement in the process of treatment and trying to be clear about a shared purpose. It also involves accepting that a child with ARFID, in particular, may initially not be strongly motivated to make any changes and to try to work positively to reassure them about the pace and direction of change. It can mean that the focus of treatment is influenced by what is going to make a meaningful change for the individual concerned. For example, a teenager with ARFID may benefit more from being able to eat socially acceptable and readily available foods, such as chips or pizza, than working on fruit and vegetables. It can in some cases be more helpful to try to add in a smoothie or a multi-vitamin and mineral supplement whilst working on socially useful foods so that age-appropriate social activities and development do not suffer. At the end of treatment, clinicians should ideally check with you whether there have been improvements in the concerns you raised at the start, and in the areas of negative impact you identified. Without such improvements, it may be hard to judge treatment as having been effective and helpful.

The second pillar of evidence-based practice is represented by 'clinical expertise'. People usually seek help for difficulties from professionals they believe hold more knowledge about what best to do and know how to access or implement the input and support required. Clinical expertise results from a combination of specialist training and the experience of both the individual practitioner as well as others working in a particular field. Individual clinical practitioners gain experience over time about a wide range of aspects of what their patients bring to them; particular patterns of difficulties and presenting symptoms; what generally works best under which circumstances; aspects of someone's life that might cause disruption or difficulty during treatment; diagnoses that might present in a similar way but need very different treatment approaches; and much more. However, if only the most experienced clinicians were any good, we would all be in trouble! This is certainly not the case as all clinical practitioners, from those who are newly qualified to those approaching retirement, are required to remain updated on developments and practices in their particular field. Fulfilling this requirement is usually an integral part of their licence to practice being renewed and one of the reasons why there are so many conferences and training workshops for clinical practitioners. The sharing of clinical expertise is a main function of such events, with the intention that this can then benefit patient care through ensuring that clinicians are up-to-date and knowledgeable.

There is no doubt that clinical expertise in relation to ARFID is accumulating. It does take a while for any new diagnostic term to 'bed down' and become part of everyone's conscious awareness. This goes for clinicians as well as the general public. At the time you read this book, ARFID should be a term recognised by the majority of clinicians working in the eating disorders field. It is also likely to be known to people working in the paediatric feeding disorders field. It is possible that not all family doctors may be aware of the term, and perhaps even likely that some specialist practitioners, for example, dermatologists, ophthalmologists, or others who do not focus on nutrition or growth, will not have much knowledge of it. Clearly, if this second pillar of clinical expertise is genuinely to form an aspect of best treatment, clinical expertise in relation to ARFID needs to be held by members of the treating team. This might mean that in some instances, parents will need to request or seek out referral to appropriate services. This can depend on local care arrangements but as some parents have described that they have had to do this, it seems worth a mention here. Whether that is a service seeing primarily young

Table 6.1 Clinical expertise informed practice: addressing the main driver(s) of avoidance/restriction

Low interest in food or eating	Sensory-based avoidance	Concern about aversive consequences
Psychoeducation	Psychoeducation	Psychoeducation
Structure/routine	Sensory diet	Graded exposure
Learning/habit acquisition	Desensitisation	Cognitive Behavioural Therapy
Arousal regulation/ attention	Disgust management strategies	Anxiety management strategies
Family interventions	Family interventions	Family interventions

people with eating disorders, or whether it is a feeding disorder service, matters less than whether staff members are informed and knowledgeable about ARFID.

What do we know from accumulated clinical expertise so far? We know that 'best treatment' is generally treatment that targets whatever is driving and maintaining the child's difficulties and addresses any acute risk. We also know that there are three commonly identified drivers of avoidance or restriction that can occur singly or in combination. Table 6.1 sets out some of the strategies and approaches that have emerged as helpful in terms of targeting drivers and maintaining factors. This table lists the three most common features underlying the eating difficulty and then under each heading, lists potentially useful approaches to try to resolve or improve matters.

You will notice that each column starts with 'psychoeducation'. This is a somewhat inelegant term for something that is vital to optimal treatment. Essentially it refers to the practice of providing all those involved in treatment, that is the child, parents/carers, siblings, and other family members as appropriate, with information about a disorder or condition, in this case anything related to ARFID; about treatment options; and about likely outcomes. Clear information can be extremely helpful, as in the case of Mohammed:

Mohammed, an eight-year-old boy developed a significant fear of choking after witnessing his aunt choke on a chicken bone during a family dinner. She had not suffered any untoward effect, but Mohammed had since become increasingly anxious and distressed at every mealtime, to the extent that eventually he would only accept liquids. Aside from being a worrier generally, there had been no other developmental concerns of note. It was decided that Mohammed might benefit from some CBT (cognitive behavioural therapy)-based sessions to help with his fear and associated avoidance behaviour. His parents were in agreement with this, and willing to work with the team by supporting Mohammed at home with his treatment homework tasks between sessions. Before starting the treatment, the Speech and Language Therapist met with Mohammed to explain how humans swallow and to go over the body's automatic responses, like coughing, that can help the swallow to correct itself when needed. She demonstrated some aspects of swallowing in the room and encouraged Mohammed to copy her. Together they looked at some videos of what happens when you swallow. Mohammed was interested and asked questions. He was then asked to tell his parents, who later joined them in the room, what he had learned. They too had an opportunity to ask questions, allowing the family to acquire a shared understanding of swallowing and normal strategies to reduce any risk of choking, such as chewing food properly and clearing one mouthful before the next. Mohammed was able to understand that limiting himself to liquids was not necessary to make sure he was safe, but he said he still felt anxious about the thought of putting anything hard or lumpy in his mouth. The psychoeducation session was important in providing factual information that helped Mohammed engage actively in the CBT sessions that followed.

Any information should be presented in an accessible way that is appropriately tailored to the understanding of the recipient. For example, a seven-year-old will need a different kind of conversation to an adult. Those directly involved in treatment alongside the clinician, at a minimum the parents and the child, need to understand what is involved and why, as well as needing to be in a position to make informed choices about next steps. For the majority of children and adolescents, parents will do this together with the child if the latter is old and able enough, or in the case of younger or less able young people, on behalf of their child. No one can be expected to make decisions if they do not know enough about the situation and the available options. Psychoeducation is therefore used to increase knowledge to enable informed decision making and to increase understanding.

You will also notice that each of the three columns in Table 6.1 ends with 'family interventions'. This is because in this book we are primarily discussing treatment for children and young people, most of whom will be living with one or more parents or caregivers. When a child or young person has ARFID, it is unusual for this not to have at least some effect on all members of the family, which might need discussion and consideration. Family interventions may include sessions with the parents alone, with the parents and the child or with the wider family. There is no hard and fast rule about this, but it is wise to keep the objective of trying to address how best to manage whatever is driving or maintaining the avoidance or restriction, as well as how best to manage the impact of this on others as the focus for family interventions. Parents will often need to implement strategies at home and so may find time without the child to talk things over with the clinician useful. If a child is engaged in some one-to-one sessions with a therapist, parents should ideally be involved in some way to be able to support their child between sessions and to be able to ensure consistency and continuity.

Sometimes family mealtimes may be offered in clinic settings. These can be helpful as an opportunity for clinicians to observe the nature and extent of eating difficulties so that they can offer the best advice and support, or to try out changes in approach or foods offered. Do remember that it is not at all uncommon for children to behave differently outside the home. In this, they are just like adults! Most of us adjust our behaviour to different circumstances and many of us like to relax and not push ourselves at home. In the same way, children may be slightly more willing to try something, for example when working with a therapist, which can then be built upon in a family mealtime in the clinic. In turn, this can help with the new behaviour being transferred to the home setting. Sometimes there can be unhelpful interactions (often unintentionally so) at the table that can be reconsidered together and modified. There are multiple potential benefits of family mealtimes in clinic, which can form a useful type of family intervention.

Turning now to the approaches listed under the 'low interest' heading in Table 6.1, you will see three key strategies listed. These are: building on structure and routine; the acquisition of learning or new habits around eating; and attending to arousal levels or the ability to pay attention. The first two are linked. We have already seen that children with this apparent lack of interest in food or eating seem not to say they are hungry and tend not to ask for food or what time meals will be. You may feel that unless you insisted, they would probably quite happily miss meals. You may have ended up in a situation where you try to make the most of any opportunity to at least get something in them, so that they don't really have a regular eating pattern in the way that others in the family have. If behaviour, in this case eating, is not initiated by the individual, we need to find some way to ensure that it happens nevertheless. Take teeth-cleaning for example. Most of us clean our teeth twice a day because it is part of our getting up and going to bed routine. It is something we were encouraged to do as children and has become a habitual behaviour to such an extent that it feels odd when we don't do it. Teeth-cleaning generally becomes a learned behaviour that we cease to stop and think about whether we will or won't do it. Under normal circumstances, eating behaviour is partly driven by hunger, but also by expectation and habit. Children with low interest in food and eating tend for a variety of reasons (discussed in Chapter 3: Why does someone develop ARFID?) not to have developed these learned behaviours and habits. Introducing clear and predictable structure in relation to mealtimes and snacks and slowly building up amounts or expectations about quantity or variety can be very helpful in supporting children with ARFID. For a child who has constantly taken the edge off any hint of appetite through eating regular small amounts, even working towards spacing slightly larger meals can help encourage hunger. Getting any child to do something that isn't top of their priorities to do at any one time can be tough, so be prepared to be calm and persistent! It takes time to acquire habits so don't lose heart if your child isn't that enthusiastic at first.

The third strategy under 'low interest' is attending to arousal levels and the ability to focus or pay attention. Many children with low interest in food or eating are more interested in other things or find it difficult to settle and focus long enough to sit and eat a meal because they want to get back to something else, or because there is too much noise or movement in the room. Such children may have high levels of distractibility, be very sensitive to environmental stimuli, or they may have significant attention problems such as in ADHD (attention deficit hyperactivity disorder). Being aware of and moderating distractions or stimuli can be helpful, but this will usually need to be combined with the strategies described above in relation to working on structure and routine. Children with ARFID generally need to know as far as is possible what is expected of them. Again, this will require persistence and time. Be prepared to start with very small changes and build up as this can sometimes be more likely to be met with success than trying to implement major changes. As always, try to notice even tiny positive steps and let your child know you have noticed in whatever way seems most appropriate – we know that this is the best way to encourage positive behaviours to develop.

Just as some children may be distracted by too many other things going on, other children actually need something additional to distract them so that they can manage to eat. Such children may often also have autism or a developmental disability. They may need to look at something or listen to something at mealtimes to ensure they eat anything. This may be watching something on a tablet, listening to music, or listening to a story or rhymes. Some children like the same thing over and over, which then becomes associated with mealtimes. When this level of distraction is needed, it is often best if it takes place at the table, or wherever the family normally eat, to maintain as far as possible at least part of the social aspect of eating as well as a link between mealtimes and a particular location where eating takes place. This may sound odd, as many parents prefer not to have electronic devices or books at the table. However, if your child needs such supports, you will know that this can really help them to eat enough, and to do so without the major battles that would otherwise ensue if you insisted they managed without. Children like this may simply not be able to tolerate a single focus on sitting and putting food into their mouth. They may need distraction, usually in the form of something familiar; the repetitive nature of this can have a centring and calming effect. Nevertheless, most normally developing children do not need this and most parents will quite appropriately discourage the regular use of devices and distractions at the table as they encourage and promote improved eating behaviour.

Let us turn now to the second column in Table 6.1, sensory based avoidance. Here again, three strategies are listed that have been shown to be helpful with children who are avoiding foods on the basis of their texture, colour, shape, appearance, minor variation in taste, temperature, smell, or other sensory property of the food in question. These are the children who may be adamant that they will only eat specific brands of foods, or will only accept food from particular places. They may need things to be presented in highly specific ways and refuse anything that does not look right. They are not inclined to take 'risks' to see if they like something or not, and are generally quite resistant to any attempts to encourage them to do so. Often they exhibit a strong disgust response when faced with food outside their preferred repertoire. Some may not be able to tolerate eating with others. Three useful strategies to consider here are the use of a 'sensory diet', desensitisation, and disgust management strategies.

A sensory diet is not a diet in the sense of foods that are eaten, it is the name given to a programme of activities that may be recommended for a particular individual, to assist with their ability to manage sensory input. The components of a sensory diet are usually put together by an occupational therapist, or other practitioner who has training and expertise in the area of sensory integration and adaptive responses to sensory input. The majority of us manage daily sensory input without too much difficulty, although we all sometimes struggle with extremes of odour, noise, brightness, etc. Some children with ARFID have heightened sensitivities; they can be regarded as 'super tasters' or 'super sensers'. If they put something unexpected or different into their mouth, they may have a very strong response to this; they may experience it as very different indeed, often combined with a sense of disgust. For some children, careful use of a tailored sensory diet can assist in dampening this response a bit, which can allow small steps forward. Sensory diets can also be helpful in children who have low interest in food and eating, in particular to assist children who are highly stimulated to become calmer and therefore manage eating slightly better. Jodie is a child who managed much better with some attention to sensory processing:

> Jodie had been struggling to eat very much at school, finding it difficult to settle and sit still. When she did manage to eat anything she seemed to have very strong reactions to it. She managed a little better at home, but her parents described her as fidgety and super-sensitive. The occupational therapist in the clinic assessed Jodie and felt that she might benefit from some strategies to help lower her arousal and also to see if it helped to diminish her extreme sensory responses. She drew up a personalised programme that Jodie's parents and her teacher could implement to see if this helped. At home, Jodie's parents were advised to try some activities before meal and snack times. These included putting one hand on each of her shoulders and pressing down, holding this for a few seconds and then repeating a number of times. They also tried bear hugs before sitting at the table, where they held Jodie and squeezed tight for a few seconds, again repeating a few times. Jodie very much enjoyed this. At school her teacher was asked if she could give Jodie some small jobs to do in the classroom, again before mealtimes. These included collecting up and carrying books, pulling open a heavy door to let the other children out, and helping to carry chairs. Again, Jodie liked being asked to do these jobs. The combination of pressure and 'heavy' work seemed to really help Jodie be able to manage mealtimes much better.

Desensitisation is a tried and tested approach to managing a person's refusal or avoidance behaviours across multiple domains. It is a relatively commonly used technique that usually follows a gradual process of exposing someone to something they have a negative response to, combined with some strategies for managing their own response. Typically a hierarchy is constructed, starting with something that does not feel too difficult to manage, working up to things that are more challenging. Two main benefits tend to be seen in children with ARFID when this technique is appropriately used. Firstly, the impact of their sensory response tends to diminish and secondly, with the addition of psychoeducation and specific disgust management strategies, children can usually learn to tolerate different foods. When introducing a new food, families are often advised to try only a very small amount on a number of consecutive days. They might be informed that only after repeated 'exposures' like this, will the child be able to decide if they might like the food or not. This is because there is an expectation that there will be a strong sensory response to anything tried for the first time. In ARFID this will very commonly be experienced as negative. With repeated tries over subsequent days, the shock of the new sensation tends to reduce, so that the child can get a better idea whether this might be something they feel able to eat or not. What typically happens is that children may be offered something new to try, they reluctantly take a taste, experience it as a shock, and then decide they are never going to try it again. Preparing the child and parents for the need to consider carefully what to try, and then to commit to daily repeated exposures to remove the effect of the initial shock, can be very helpful.

In relation to managing sensory-based avoidance, strategies to manage disgust can also be helpful. Disgust can be viewed as a helpful human response to things that might cause harm, and in this way is part of a normal repertoire of responses. In children with ARFID, many foods and aspects of eating seem to elicit extreme disgust. The task is not to completely remove this, but to reduce it and make it more manageable. Again, in part, this will come through getting used to something new, but it might also need some specific attention. Clinical experience suggests that helpful ways to do this are to combine offering an explanation to improve understanding of why the child might respond with spitting out and further rejection, and to use core cognitive behavioural techniques to help the child (where possible) and parents recognise automatic negative assumptions and to conduct experiments to demonstrate changes in disgust response. This is slightly different from traditional desensitisation therapy for fears and phobias, where the typical management strategy is to use relaxation or other anxiety reducing techniques. Disgust and fear are different human emotions which need slightly different approaches.

The third and final column in Table 6.1 lists some of the strategies that we know from clinical experience can be helpful in children where the avoidance or restriction of food and eating is driven or maintained by concern or fear about aversive consequences. These are in many respects not dissimilar from what has been discussed above, but more closely resemble standard approaches to anxiety presentations. Anxiety disorders, which include a range of difficulties such as specific phobias, separation anxiety, generalised anxiety, and social anxiety, have consistently been shown to respond well to cognitive behavioural interventions. Some form of CBT is therefore usually recommended as a first line psychological treatment for anxiety, including the use of CBT techniques delivered by parents in the case of younger or less able children. Graded exposure may form part of CBT, which in the case of anxiety is typically linked with developing skills to tolerate and eventually lower the fear response. Again, fear is a normal human response to perceived threat or danger and not something that anyone would aim to take away completely. The goal of psychological interventions for troublesome anxiety, that is anxiety that is adversely affecting behaviour, day-to-day functioning and someone's quality of life, is to help them recognise situations that cause anxiety, recognise what happens when they are anxious, and to equip them with skills to reduce the impact and intensity of feeling anxious.

In ARFID, fear-based avoidance or restriction of eating can similarly be effectively treated through using basic CBT principles, supported by appropriate involvement of parents in the case of most children and young people. Food chaining techniques, where different but similar foods may be offered can be helpful in terms of working up a hierarchy of difficulty. An example might be offering a child who accepts one type of milk chocolate chip biscuit another brand or a biscuit with white chocolate chips. The new biscuit is broadly similar but will be different to the child. If this is accepted, another new food can be added with something else changed, for example a chocolate chip cake. In this way it is possible both to build on what the child already eats, but also to allow the child's confidence about varying their diet to grow. It can be attempted with most things, for example moving from chips, to potato waffles, or other similar potato products. Although from a nutritional perspective, the new foods might not add much, this technique can help greatly with willingness to try new foods and often represents a useful start.

Until now, in our discussion of the second pillar of evidence-based practice, we have primarily addressed what clinical expertise tells us about helpful emotional, behavioural, sensory and arousal based treatment approaches. Clearly children with ARFID also often have physical treatment needs, including nutritional interventions and medical management of the impact of energy or nutritional deficiencies. A dietitian may be involved in providing advice about how best to boost your child's overall nutrition through the use of supplements. This may range from over-the-counter supplements, such as the vitamin and mineral liquids, tablets, and chewables that you can find in many supermarkets, to prescribed preparations that contain a comprehensive mix of essential nutrients and/or act to increase overall calorie intake. Dietetic advice can be extremely helpful as children have differing needs and some specialist knowledge may be required, particularly in children with ARFID who may struggle more than most other children to take the supplement in the first place, due to its taste, texture or general difference from what they might usually have. Often dietetic advice may need some additional support to achieve successful implementation. In the same way as the introduction of new foods was discussed using a hierarchy and gradual exposure above, these techniques might also be needed to help children accept a supplement.

Some children may require a period of tube feeding to help correct acute nutritional deficits if all attempts to encourage them to eat enough by mouth have failed. This may initially be via a nasogastric tube, which is a special fine tube that is inserted up through the nose and goes down the oesophagus into the stomach. This is only usually needed if the child is very unwell and will only be undertaken under medical supervision. Feeding via nasogastric tube is usually only intended as a short-term measure and generally should not last longer than a few months at the most. The child is then fed specially prepared nutritional feeds via the tube, often as a top-up to what they are taking orally. Mostly these are liquid feeds that can either be taken orally or via a tube. The doctor or dietitian will advise on the most appropriate feed. A small number of children are fed via the tube with blended foods, however these need to be specially prepared according to careful recipes and need to be extremely finely blended so that they do not block the tube. Most families do not possess a suitable blender and the practice is generally considered somewhat controversial. It can also be difficult to ensure all the necessary nutrients are present in the feed. One downside of prolonged nasogastric feeding of any kind is that it can put children off eating and drinking by mouth.

Some children with ARFID present for treatment with a tube in place. This may either be a nasogastric tube, as mentioned above, or it may be a gastrostomy tube, or in a few cases, a jejunostomy tube. Feeding via one of these tubes is sometimes referred to as 'enteral feeding'. A gastrostomy tube is inserted surgically into the stomach wall and so allows feed to be administered directly to the stomach. This type of tube may be placed if attempts to move the child to adequate oral feeding from a nasogastric tube have not been successful; if the likely pace of change is very slow and there is an increased risk that prolonged nasogastric feeding will reduce interest in oral feeding; or if gastrostomy feeding was originally required in relation to another medical condition, now resolved, but the child has failed to progress to adequate oral feeding because of avoidance or restriction typical of ARFID. Jejunostomy feeding is not usually required but in extreme cases, often associated with persistent vomiting, a tube may be surgically inserted directly into the jejunum, which is the part of the small intestine where most nutrients from food are absorbed. If tube feeding is technically not required for medical reasons, with the main reason it continues being the child failing to take enough by mouth because of avoidance or restriction, then helping reduce dependency on the tube is likely to be a major focus for treatment. This is sometimes called 'tube weaning'. You may recall the case of John in Chapter 4, when we discussed possible *consequences* of having ARFID.

John had become dependent on being fed via the jejunostomy tube. He was completely stuck in needing to exert strict control over his intake and was terrified of eating anything. However, he had been able to start taking very small amounts of two or three smooth, soft foods, and was able put single squares of chocolate into his mouth, allowing these to melt. John was upset about not being able to eat and fearful that he would stay this way for the rest of his life. He missed some of the meals he had previously enjoyed. His parents were also extremely anxious about making any changes as John had been so unwell that they thought they might lose him. The family appeared helpless and life revolved around tube feeding.

Treatment involved individual sessions for John, to work on identifying the detail of what was driving his anxiety and helping him to manage this; sessions for his parents, to help them with their own anxiety about John and to support them in encouraging him to make some changes; and some sessions for the whole family, to practice new strategies to be able to manage an initial transition back to gastrostomy feeding and subsequently to eating by mouth. John's treatment took a long time and a lot of hard work by all involved. Progress was initially very slow, but through being consistent and slowly but surely increasing the amounts and types of food John was taking by mouth, it was possible to gradually decrease the amount of feed going via the tube. Eventually he managed to successfully cease to need to be fed anything via the tube. After having maintained his weight and eating for three months, the tube was removed. The family celebrated with a weekend trip to the coast where John was able to enjoy fish and chips on the beach.

Tube weaning is essentially a process of increasing intake of food and fluid by mouth instead of feed going through a tube. A lot of the techniques listed in Table 6.1 and discussed above may be appropriate to assist with increasing intake. As we have seen in Chapter 3 (Why does someone develop ARFID?), children who have had long-term tube feeding may not develop a good sense of hunger and may therefore show low interest in food or eating. Similarly, if the child has an anxious temperament and they are not used to eating very much or a good range of foods, they may be nervous about increasing the amount or range that they eat. If they have needed a tube because of a distressing incident or medical condition, they might be fearful that this might re-occur. Some children with significant sensory sensitivities, including children with autism, may have required tube feeding due to rejection of most tastes and textures. Once tube feeding has become established, it can be very hard to encourage change due to the sensory challenges that go along with eating. As with any aspect of ARFID, it is important to be realistic about change, both in terms of what may be achieved and what a 'good enough' diet would look like. Some children with developmental delays may not have the oral-motor development and functional skills to be able to manage the same types of food as their peers; soft and pureed foods may represent the most appropriate texture for them in terms of their capabilities and capacity to manage food. Helping children away from tube dependency when medically they should be able to manage without, is invariably in a child's best interests.

We can now turn to the third and final pillar of evidence-based practice, that is, information obtained through clinically relevant, well conducted, well designed research studies. Perhaps unsurprisingly, given the recent introduction of ARFID, this will be the shortest section. A couple of things deserve mention. Firstly, there are plenty of good research studies that we can learn from, involving people with conditions that seem related to ARFID, such as anxiety and other feeding difficulties. However, at present there are very few studies specifically testing treatments with people formally diagnosed as having ARFID. Secondly, any recommendations for the use of medication specifically for the treatment of ARFID should be based on trials involving people with that diagnosis. Thirdly, there is currently a significant amount of research interest into possible treatments for ARFID, meaning that this spindly pillar is likely to become more substantial as time goes by. Early studies testing how helpful CBT and family-based interventions can be in the treatment of ARFID have shown that both these approaches can be helpful for some individuals and families. This is reassuring as the findings are broadly consistent with practice informed by clinical expertise. However, we remain a long way off having good evidence to support exactly what form of treatment is best for which individuals. The third pillar therefore continues very much to need the additional support of the other two pillars of patient values and clinical expertise.

In relation to medication, there is, as yet, no evidence to support the use of medication as a preferred treatment for ARFID itself. Some medicines may undoubtedly prove helpful as a supportive treatment, but only after the main strategies such as managing acute weight and growth issues, addressing nutritional deficiencies, and using psychological, family and sensory interventions to address avoidance or restriction, have been attempted. If any medication is recommended for your child, it is always worth checking how it is understood to help. Of course, some children with ARFID may be prescribed medication for co-occurring conditions. One aspect of this that can cause concern is the use of ADHD medication in children with both ARFID and ADHD. This is because the use of these medications has been found to be associated with appetite loss. If you have a child with ADHD who has low interest in eating, the prospect of further loss of appetite may be a worry. However, clinical experience often shows that the improvement in focus and attention that occurs through taking the medication can facilitate eating in some of these children with ADHD and ARFID. In such situations, the use of ADHD medication can therefore be extremely helpful. Other medications that may be suggested are cyproheptadine, an anti-histamine, or in some cases, low doses of olanzapine, an anti-psychotic. There is some emerging evidence to suggest that these medications may prove helpful in some individuals, but always only as a supportive intervention alongside other treatment approaches.

In this chapter we have considered how to answer the question 'What is the best treatment for ARFID?' It seems very unlikely that one treatment approach will be best for all, due to the complexities and variability in features of ARFID as well as differences in its impact across different individuals and families. 'Best' treatment is therefore likely to be treatment that is tailored to the needs and requirements of the particular child and family, and should be relevant to them. One final note of caution; it is wise to avoid 'over-treatment'. Far better to concentrate on achieving a modest level of change that is meaningful, reduces risk, and enables the child to improve their psychological and social functioning, than to keep going with appointments for prolonged periods so that they lose motivation and food and eating become over-emphasised. Over-treatment can also occur when the child might have 'good enough' growth and a 'good enough' diet despite having a fairly restricted or limited intake, when that intake is not having an adverse impact on their development or day-to-day functioning. Sometimes an over-focus on pushing children to eat a wider range or eat more food, when this is not really necessary for the child to thrive, ends up making food more of a battle ground than it needs to be. Children who are cautious eaters may become more adventurous with their eating as they grow older, or if they don't, they may develop greater awareness that their eating is beginning to be a problem for them and the beginnings of a wish for things to be different. Intervening when some awareness of difficulty, and some motivation to explore the possibility of making changes are in place, is likely to be much more productive. Best treatment therefore also includes an element of ensuring the timing is right.

Chapter 7

What about the future?

One very common question asked by parents is whether their child is at greater risk of developing an eating disorder like anorexia nervosa or bulimia nervosa, because they have had ARFID. Others worry that their child may suffer lasting negative effects in terms of their physical health or growth, due to their limited diet. Some parents wonder whether the child's siblings will also develop ARFID. When you are struggling to manage a child's eating, these and other concerns about longer-term outcomes are understandable. It can be very difficult to see the light at the end of the tunnel when daily battles about what is and what isn't eaten seem to dominate family life. Questions and concerns tend to pop up and multiply. They can linger and become difficult to banish, despite best attempts to do so.

This final chapter is therefore about how best to address questions and concerns like these, through discussing what is known about course and outcome in relation to ARFID. *Course* is the last of our 'C' factors. The chapter includes a summary of the evidence about what happens to children who have been given a diagnosis of ARFID, as well as what is known about the outcomes for children whose eating habits resemble an ARFID presentation. We will consider what is known about factors that have been identified as having a positive or a negative influence on the course of ARFID. We will also consider some of the wider issues previously referred to, like anxiety and autism, and reflect on their relationship to what might happen in the future.

To start us off, let's get some terms clear. When we think about the *course* of any illness or disorder, it can be helpful to use the analogy of a pathway. Some people define the start of the pathway as the time of diagnosis and the end of the pathway as recovery. In ARFID these two time points can be somewhat tricky to determine. If your child has very longstanding feeding difficulties, it might be hard to pinpoint a specific time at which being picky or fussy became more extreme and tipped into ARFID. It can be more straightforward to determine the start of the pathway if your child has a more sudden onset of difficulties, for example in the cases of a choking incident like in Emmie's situation (in Chapter 1), or a distressing experience like in Jake's (Chapter 1), or Lewis's (Chapter 3). In these instances you might be able to more confidently identify a specific point in time when the difficulties became significant and concerning. In general it seems most helpful to think of the start of the ARFID pathway as when you noticed that your child's eating behaviour was definitely different to their peers', when it began to interfere with day-to-day life, or when you noticed that they seemed to be struggling physically because of their restricted diet. In reality, this may be a long time before a formal diagnosis is made.

If this is the starting point for the course of the disorder, how do we define the endpoint? Put another way, how should 'recovery' from ARFID be defined? This remains a subject for discussion amongst clinicians and researchers, with as yet no clear consensus. However, a couple of things seem evident. Firstly, that recovery might look different in different people and secondly that what is regarded as a good outcome might not constitute full recovery. Technically, someone no longer has ARFID if they no longer meet diagnostic criteria. Yet that is often not a very helpful way to look at things, as some aspects of the problem may linger and continue to cause some disruption to daily life. Your child may have progressed to a 'good enough' diet and their weight and growth may be satisfactory, but there might still be some mealtime battles or restrictions on what you can do as family. Some parents might settle for this, knowing how far things have come, while others may feel that this remains unsatisfactory and want to continue to work on making improvements. Essentially, aiming for complete eradication of any avoidance or restriction in relation to eating behaviour may be unrealistic; after all, the majority of people have some things they don't like to eat, or amounts they feel uncomfortable with. A more meaningful goal might be to arrive at a point where any avoidance or restriction is manageable, and it does not have an undue adverse effect on your child's health or development, their day-to-day functioning, or your family life.

Let's now turn to what research studies can tell us about course and outcome. As with so many aspects of ARFID, our knowledge based on the results of formal research studies remains limited. As we have seen, this is only to be expected, given the relatively recent introduction of the term ARFID. What seems to be emerging is that positive outcomes can certainly be achieved as long as treatment focusses on the things that matter most. That might sound obvious, but because ARFID is a term that covers a number of different types of eating difficulty, sometimes there might be a misplaced focus on a less important detail for any one individual. For example, we have seen in Chapter 6 that it can sometimes be very helpful to focus on introducing a socially useful food, for example, fries or chips, rather than something like a banana or green vegetables. If a child is taking a vitamin and mineral supplement, nutritional risk may be managed in a way similar to applying a sticking plaster. Being able to manage eating out, even if it is only chips, may help with self-confidence and social interaction which is important. In turn, these things may lead eventually to being able to take more challenging steps with eating, ideally to include foods to help the overall nutritional balance of accepted foods, like bananas or greens. Starting with these might simply lead to feelings of failure and increased resistance from the child.

Another clear example is an emphasis on weight gain, where this is not the most pressing problem. Some children with ARFID may be quite slim and have always been so. On balance, this may not be the most immediately concerning aspect of their presentation. If treatment solely focusses on the need to take in more calories to gain weight, it is unlikely to help other possibly more problematic aspects of the individual's difficulty, such as an inability to widen their range. Such misplaced emphases may in some instances inadvertently prolong difficulties.

Fortunately, we do know that appropriately directed management can be very effective in terms of reducing risk and improving outcomes. Clinical evidence certainly points to better outcomes when careful assessment has been used to identify the specific drivers and hurdles present in any one individual, which can then be targeted. Children with very low weights can be helped to gain weight; those with dangerously narrow diets can be helped to expand them so that their basic nutritional needs are covered; and children who have been unable to participate in age appropriate activities can be supported to join in, often through making relatively small changes to their eating behaviour.

A key consideration here is the matter of expectations. It is vital to make sure these are realistic. Does a good outcome mean that your child will enthusiastically sit down and tuck into a full Sunday roast with all the trimmings when they have existed on pasta shapes and chocolate pots for years? Or does a good outcome mean that your child can usually participate in a family meal, but still requires some low key encouragement and continues to have some things they decline? Is a good outcome being able to go to any restaurant and pick the most exotic thing from the menu, or is a good outcome being able to visit a handful of restaurants and sticking to the same 'safe' but commonly available dishes? Different families tend to have different expectations, which may be a reflection of lifestyle and family values just as much as the level of desire to achieve change.

We asked a number of parents attending our clinic what they hoped might be achieved by attending and receiving treatment for their child's ARFID. Most were modest and realistic about their expectations. Here are some examples of what parents typically wanted for their children:

- to be able to eat bigger helpings
- to enjoy food more
- to have more variety in their diet
- to stop being anxious around food
- to be willing to try new foods

- not to need tube feeding
- not to need supplement drinks
- to start to manage lumps and textures
- to feed him/herself
- to eat more quickly

and for their families:

- to be able to go out to eat as a family
- to have normal family mealtimes.

Achieving these things would represent a good outcome for many of these parents, at least in terms of what they hoped to achieve by the end of a period of work in the clinic. Some of these things may seem relevant to your own situation. The ability to determine whether such goals are achieved, varies somewhat. No longer needing a tube is easier to be clear about than increasing enjoyment or decreasing anxiety. In order to decide if emotional changes have been achieved, we are often reliant on observing the child's behaviour. Older children and adolescents may of course be able to express their emotions and changes in how they feel about food, but with many younger children, or those with delayed development, we may need to rely on how they behave around food to decide if there is more enjoyment or less anxiety. Similarly, the concept of a 'normal' family mealtime is not precisely defined, making the objective measurement of how many families achieve this quite challenging.

The best judges of outcome of treatment are of course families themselves. However, as we have seen, what one family hopes for may be different to another. This is not solely due to the specifics of the child's feeding or eating difficulties, but due to differences in the impact of these on the child's life and on family life, differences in expectations, differences in family values, and differences in levels of available support. Remaining positive, noticing efforts made by your child, reminding them of changes they have successfully made, even if these may seem tiny, are very important in keeping movement along the pathway going in the right direction.

These are active, helpful things that parents can do to assist with increasing the likelihood of good progress and positive outcomes.

All of this has a bearing on formal outcome research. Most studies investigating the outcomes of illnesses, medical conditions or disorders, tend to use markers of good outcome decided by clinicians. For example, from an orthopaedic surgeon's point of view, a good outcome of surgical intervention to realign a broken tibia might be a well healed leg which allows the patient to bear their own weight. From the patient's perspective a good outcome might be being able to get on their bicycle again. In research studies of patients undergoing tibia repair surgery, it is far more likely that data would be gathered on the basis of measurements of bone realignment than data about how many patients are cycling. You can see that with something like ARFID, outcome research could be complicated! Of course it is possible to report on success in terms of weight gain, growth, or the nutritional adequacy of diets, but these are only part of the picture.

There are a number of studies that have shown that older children and adolescents, most commonly with recent onset types of ARFID (e.g. those who have restricted their eating after a distressing event such as choking), who have lost a lot of weight, can be successfully helped to regain weight and supported to maintain their improved weight status. Obviously this is important, but it does not tell us a great deal about the impact of ARFID more generally and whether this has been alleviated. There has also been some suggestion that within this particular ARFID population, a few may go on to develop anorexia nervosa. It is very important to note that it is extremely difficult to be clear whether this might be because they have been misdiagnosed in the first place, or whether this is indeed one possible pathway for a small number of people.

Let's try to unpick this issue in a bit more detail, not least because it is often on parents' minds. At present, there is insufficient evidence to support the notion that ARFID increases the risk of later development of anorexia nervosa or bulimia nervosa. This statement is true in general terms, in other words, it is true at a population level. This does not necessarily mean that any one person who has had ARFID will never develop an eating disorder later. It means that there is no evidence to show that children who have had ARFID (of any type) are, as a group, clearly at greater risk of later development of an eating disorder. In fact there is more evidence to show that certain variants of ARFID might persist in a more stable form over time rather than change into another eating disorder. The clearest evidence in this respect relates to children with low interest in eating and those with sensory based avoidance.

So if there is no clear evidence of a direct pathway between ARFID and anorexia nervosa or bulimia nervosa, why might this sometimes happen? One finding that has emerged fairly clearly from research is that mealtime conflict – that is arguments about food and eating at the table, or stressful interactions over meals – is not at all helpful. In fact, it has been proposed that it is mealtime conflict that can raise the risk of later development of an eating disorder. In the clinic, we will often advise parents of children with ARFID to be aware of this, and to limit conflict at the table. It is not hard to understand that if mealtimes are always unpleasant and difficult, with rowing and children feeling under pressure to eat things they feel unable to, the whole arena of eating becomes quite sensitive. Anorexia nervosa is a complex disorder but the individual exerting control over their food intake is an important part of it. It may be that conflict in the face of the child with ARFID's genuine difficulty with eating increases their need to exert control? The precise mechanisms are a long way from being understood but the take-home message of limiting mealtime conflict as far as possible seems important in terms of longer-term outcomes.

A number of other aspects of a child's temperament, health, general functioning, and wider development may also have a bearing on course and outcome. For example, a child with an anxious temperament may go through a number of different manifestations of anxiety if they find themselves in stressful or difficult situations. They may experience difficulties separating when starting playgroup or school, they may be very shy, or they may have quite extreme childhood fears. Some children with ARFID are certainly temperamentally anxious. Many will have had periods of anxiety-related behavioural difficulties other than those related to eating. Some anxious children may take a long time to learn to manage their fears or worries; indeed some adults with an anxious temperament continue to find this a challenge at times. In some individuals with ARFID in the context of this type of anxiety, an initial episode may resolve but then re-occur later, typically when a newly stressful situation occurs. This is more likely if the individual concerned has not acquired the skills needed to cope with their inbuilt response to anything they perceive as anxiety provoking. In this way, anxiety can sometimes mean that ARFID might persist a little longer or tend to come back again.

We know from Chapter 2 (Who can develop ARFID?) that anxiety is one of the main *correlates* of the disorder. Other common ones are the neurodevelopmental disorders (including autism and ADHD) as well as developmental delays and disabilities. These things do not necessarily mean that the likely course and outcome of ARFID is better or worse than in children without these conditions. However, it does mean that efforts to address the difficulties need to be adapted to suit the child. Where this does not happen, then in general, outcomes are likely to be poorer. Where it does happen, children with ARFID in the context of other difficulties can make significant improvements and their eating can cease to be a primary concern.

So does ARFID in itself raise the risk of later development of other disorders, including a whole range of mental health problems? The answer is most likely not. Current evidence suggests that it is much more likely that genetic vulnerabilities combined with individual experience predispose people to a range of problems, of which ARFID may be one. In some individuals, ARFID may be *associated* with later problems rather than directly *lead to* later difficulties. In many children however, ARFID will resolve during childhood and children will mature into healthy, well-functioning adults. It is not at all unusual for some parents to tell us that they too struggled with avoidant or restrictive eating behaviour when they were younger, but the vast majority have firmly put all such difficulties behind them.

As with all disorders, a small minority of children will continue to experience significant difficulties with their eating and change may be extremely slow or feel non-existent. Some may continue to need support with their nutrition and some may encounter daily challenges in accepting food. As a minimum, it is always possible to lower risk through nutritional support and reducing distress. If there is an illness or condition with a 100% cure rate, it usually means that the cause is simple and well-known, and the treatment always effective. We are not at this point with ARFID, which as we have seen throughout this book is complicated in terms of its causes (see Chapter 3) and still lacking stand-out first line evidence-based treatments (see Chapter 6). Indeed, this complexity and degree of uncertainty may be one of the reasons you have been reading this book! However, it does mean that we still have more work to do to understand what it is that holds some children back, and to develop ways of achieving positive outcomes for as many children as possible in a safe and efficient way. The body of research on course and outcome is very limited and currently tells us rather little. This can only get better with improved recognition of ARFID and the increase in interest in trying to move effective treatments forwards.

This chapter is called 'What about the future?' It ends with some suggestions from parents about what they want from services for children with ARFID; what future services should embrace in their thinking about how they will be run. As with measurement of outcomes, all too often clinics and hospitals design services from the perspective of clinicians and managers. Thankfully, this is changing in most countries, with so-called 'patient-centred care' approaches now being much more widely championed. Essentially this means that people who use healthcare services should be much more closely involved in saying what the design and delivery of those services should look like. Above, we looked at a number of things parents attending our clinic said they wanted to achieve by the end of treatment. We asked the same parents what they thought an ideal service should look like. They made a number of very helpful practical suggestions. Here are the most frequently mentioned ones:

- Staff should help children and families to feel supported and reassured, and take children's problems seriously

- Staff should all be friendly and approachable
- Staff should be knowledgeable and have expertise in ARFID
- The team should include different types of clinicians (i.e. a multi-disciplinary team)
- There needs to be a fun/relaxing safe area where the child can play or be otherwise occupied while parents talk with clinicians
- Families should be seen promptly to minimise anxiety
- Appointments should be offered for the child together with the parents as well as for parents alone
- Time should be taken to gain a good understanding of the child's problem
- Appointments should be long enough to talk things through, e.g. one hour
- Advice should be given on what strategies can be put into place at home
- There needs to be the option of contacting the clinic to talk to someone between visits

All these requests seem perfectly reasonable and sensible. They also seem eminently do-able in terms of providing a service. It is vital that families are given the time and space to discuss the difficulties they are facing. These will differ between families and the extra time spent trying to better understand the individual child and family's situation is invariably well spent time in terms of promoting positive outcomes. Similarly the stronger the trust between families and clinicians, and the more collaborative and jointly owned the business of working together to support the child, the greater the potential for success.

Chapter 8

Closing words

It will be clear to you that this book is not a treatment manual or a simple step-by-step guide to managing your child's eating difficulties. The reason for this is very straightforward. ARFID is a complex, multi-faceted condition, which can vary in its main features across different people. At this point in time simply not enough is known about ARFID to be able to confidently recommend adopting one particular strategy or another. There is no one tried and tested treatment approach. It is too soon to be able to set out with any degree of certainty what parents and carers *should* do. What the book has set out to do is to engage in an honest, open conversation with you about the current state of knowledge about ARFID, to provide you with some ways of structuring your own assessment of different aspects of your child's eating difficulty, and to equip you with some pointers and ideas that might prove helpful in your own situation. It represents an attempt to address common questions and concerns raised by parents or carers grappling with ARFID in their child, through sharing some of the experiences of many families seen through the lens of clinical encounters. Wherever you are in your own journey, I hope that at least some of the content proves helpful.

References

American Psychiatric Association (APA) (2013) *Diagnostic and Statistical Manual of Mental Disorders*, Fifth Edition. Arlington VA: American Psychiatric Association

Bryant-Waugh, R. (2006) Pathways to recovery: Promoting change within a developmental systemic framework. *Clinical Child Psychology and Psychiatry* 11(2), 213–224

Engel, GL. (1997) The need for a new medical model: a challenge for biomedicine. *Science* 196, 129–136

Engel, GL. (1980) The clinical application of the biopsychosocial model. *American Journal of Psychiatry* 137(5), 535–544.

Sackett, DL, Rosenberg, WMC, Gray, JAM, Haynes, RB & Richardson, WS. (1996) Evidence based medicine: what it is and what it isn't. *British Medical Journal* 3(12), 71

Sackett, DL, Strauss, SE, Richardson, WS, Rosenberg, W & Haynes, RB. (2000) *Evidence-based Medicine: How to Practise and Teach EBM*, Second Edition. London: Churchill Livingstone

World Health Organization (2018) *International Statistical Classification of Diseases and Related Health Problems*, 11th Revision. Retrieved from https://icd.who.int/browse11/l-m/en

Index